MRI OF THE HAND AND WRIST

MRI OF THE HAND AND WRIST

THOMAS H. BERQUIST, M.D., F.A.C.R.

Professor of Radiology
Mayo Medical School
Director for Education
Mayo Foundation
Rochester, Minnesota
Consultant
Department of Diagnostic Radiology
Mayo Clinic Jacksonville
Jacksonville, Florida

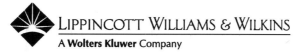

LIPPINCOTT WILLIAMS & WILKINS
A **Wolters Kluwer** Company

Philadelphia • Baltimore • New York • London
Buenos Aires • Hong Kong • Sydney • Tokyo

Acquisitions Editor: Beth Barry
Developmental Editor: Scott Scheidt
Production Editor: Karina Mikhli
Manufacturing Manager: Benjamin Rivera
Cover Designer: Christine Jenny
Compositor: TechBooks
Printer: Maple Press

Published by LIPPINCOTT WILLIAMS & WILKINS
530 Walnut Street
Philadelphia, PA 19106 USA
LWW.com

Library of Congress Cataloging-in-Publication Data

MRI of the hand and wrist / editor, Thomas H. Berquist.
    p. ; cm.
  Includes bibliographical references and index.
  ISBN 0-7817-3796-6
    1. Hand—Magnetic resonance imaging.   2. Wrist—Magnetic resonance imaging.
I. Berquist, Thomas H. (Thomas Henry), 1945–
    [DNLM: 1. Hand—radiography.   2. Magnetic Resonance Imaging—methods.
3. Wrist—radiography.   WE 830 M939 2003]
  RC951.M76   2003
  617.5'7507548—dc21
                                   2002043362

10 9 8 7 6 5 4 3 2 1

CONTENTS

CONTRIBUTING AUTHORS

Kimberly K. Amrami, M.D.   Assistant Professor of Radiology, Mayo Medical School; and Consultant, Department of Radiology, Mayo Clinic, Rochester, Minnesota

Laura Wasylenko Bancroft, M.D.   Assistant Professor of Radiology, Mayo Medical School; and Consultant, Department of Radiology, Mayo Clinic Jacksonville, Jacksonville, Florida

Thomas H. Berquist, M.D., F.A.C.R.   Professor of Radiology, Mayo Medical School; Director for Education, Mayo Foundation, Rochester, Minnesota; and Consultant, Department of Diagnostic Radiology, Mayo Clinic Jacksonville, Jacksonville, Florida

Mark J. Kransdorf, M.D.   Professor of Radiology, Mayo Medical School; and Consultant, Department of Radiology, Mayo Clinic Jacksonville, Jacksonville, Florida

Jeffrey James Peterson, M.D.   Assistant Professor of Radiology, Mayo Medical School; and Consultant, Department of Diagnostic Radiology, Mayo Clinic Jacksonville, Jacksonville, Florida

PREFACE

Clinical applications for MRI of the hand and wrist continue to expand due to improved imaging techniques, new coil technology, and the resulting fine anatomic detail provided by these upgrades. Therefore, it is now even more important that radiologists and clinicians understand the applications and limitations of MRI for evaluating hand and wrist disorders.

This text emphasizes MR anatomy, techniques, and clinical applications. Comparison of MRI with CT, ultrasound, and other imaging techniques is discussed where appropriate. Chapter 1 provides anatomic information using common MR pulse sequences, MR arthrography, and frequently used image planes. Technique is discussed in Chapter 2 to avoid redundancy in later pathologic chapters. Chapter 3 discusses common technical and anatomic pitfalls that must be understood to avoid errors in interpreting MR images. Chapters 4–10 discuss specific clinical applications for MRI of the hand and wrist; the current role of MRI, focused techniques, and comparison with other imaging modalities is also discussed.

This text provides a comprehensive reference for radiologists, residents, and physicians (emergency room physicians, rheumatologists, internists, orthopedic surgeons, sports medicine physicians, family medicine physicians, physical medicine specialists, etc.) who deal with hand and wrist disorders.

Thomas H. Berquist

ACKNOWLEDGMENTS

Preparation of this text was facilitated by Noel Bahr, Lisa Giles, and Jeannette Lynch. I wish to thank them for their support in image retrieval and in printing the numerous MR images.

Daniel Hubert from the section of Medical Photography was instrumental in providing the necessary photographs and prints of images used in this text. John Hagen, from the Department of Medical Graphics provided the superb illustrations necessary to demonstrate anatomy, specific classifications, and pathology.

The manuscript was prepared by Linda Downie and Pamela Chirico. Their hard work and orchestration efforts were greatly appreciated.

Finally, I wish to thank Beth Barry, Scott Scheidt, and Karina Mikhli of Lippincott Williams & Wilkins for their assistance in the development and production of this text.

MRI OF THE HAND AND WRIST

ANATOMY

THOMAS H. BERQUIST

Numerous imaging techniques have been employed to demonstrate the complex osseous and soft-tissue anatomy of the hand and wrist.[9,10,27] Magnetic resonance imaging (MRI) provides superior anatomic detail in multiple image planes. Therefore, knowledge of the anatomy in multiple image planes is essential for clinicians and radiologists.

OSSEOUS ANATOMY

There are 8 carpal bones in the wrist and 5 metacarpals and 14 phalanges in the hand.[4,9,16] The proximal carpal row (scaphoid, lunate, triquetrum) articulates with the distal radius and ulna (Fig. 1-1).[16]

Distal Radius

The distal radius (metaphysis and epiphysis) is primarily canallous bone with a thin cortical shell[11] and is elongated on the radial side forming the radial styloid (Figs. 1-1 and 1-2). The lateral surface of the radial styloid contains a double groove for the tendons of the first dorsal compartment (I, extensor pollicis brevis and abductor pollicis longus) (Fig. 1-2B).

The convex dorsal (posterior) surface of the distal radius contains multiple grooves for the second through fourth extensor compartments. There is a prominent ridge between the second and third compartments termed Lister's tubercle (Fig. 1-2B).[16,35] The palmar (anterior) surface of the distal radius is slightly concave and roughened for the attachments of the radiocarpal ligaments.[35]

The ulnar surface of the distal radius is termed the sigmoid fossa or ulnar notch. The semicircular notch has dorsal, palmar, and distal margins (Fig. 1-3).[16] The dorsal and palmar aspect serves for attachment of the radioulnar ligaments.

The distal radial articular surface contains two fossae for the scaphoid and lunate articulations (Fig. 1-4).[11] The distal articular surface has a normal palmar tilt of 11 to12° in the sagittal plane and a radial inclination angle of 24° in the coronal or frontal plane (Fig. 1-5).[9,11,16]

Distal Ulna

The enlarged end of the ulna (ulnar head) articulates with the sigmoid notch of the distal radius and the lunate and triquetrum distally (Fig. 1-6).[35] The distal ulna consists of three distinct portions: (a) the semicircular articular surface of articular cartilage adjacent to the triangular fibrocartilage; (b) a rough central depression for attachment of the triangular fibrocartilage; and (c) a medial prominence termed the ulnar styloid.[16,35] There is a groove in the dorsal (posterior) ulna for the sixth dorsal compartment (extensor carpi ulnaris) (Fig. 1-6).[16,35] The ulna and radius may vary in length at the radioulnar articulation. When the ulna is longer, it is termed ulnar positive variance and when shorter, ulnar negative variance (Fig. 1-7).[1,16,34]

Scaphoid

The scaphoid is the largest carpal bone in the proximal row and serves as an important link between the proximal and distal carpal rows.[16,35,36] The scaphoid articulates with the radius, the lunate medially, the capitate distomedially, and the trapezium and trapezoid distally (Fig. 1-8).[11,35,38]

There is a tuberosity on the distal palmar aspect for ligament attachments. The scaphoid ridge or waist is located on the mid-lateral surface and accepts about 80% of the vascular supply for the scaphoid (Fig. 1-8).[16,35]

Lunate

The lunate is rectangular in the coronal plane and "moon shaped" in the sagittal plane (Fig. 1-9). About 80% of the surface is covered by articular cartilage. The lunate has four articular surfaces for the radius proximally, scaphoid laterally, triquetrum medially, and capitate and lunate distally. There are palmar and dorsal nonarticular surfaces. Viegas et al.[44] described the lunate as type 1 or 2, based on the articulation with the hamate (Fig. 1-10). Type 1 (34.5%) has no hamate articulation and type 2 (65.5%) contains a hamate articular facet. The articular facet for the capitate is larger than the hamate in 65% of patients.[16]

The lunate may also be classified by surface configuration in relation to the radius, ulna, and triangular fibrocartilage

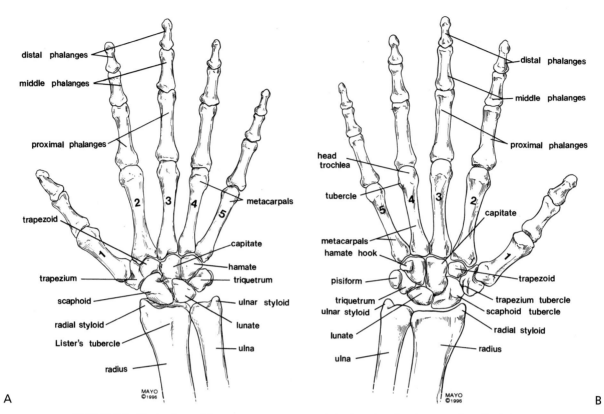

FIGURE 1-1. Illustration of the osseous structures of the hand and wrist seen dorsally **(A)** and from the palmar surface **(B)**. (From Berger RA. General anatomy. In: Cooney WP III, Linscheid RL, Dobyns JH, eds. The wrist: diagnosis and operative treatment. St. Louis: Mosby, 1998:32–60.)

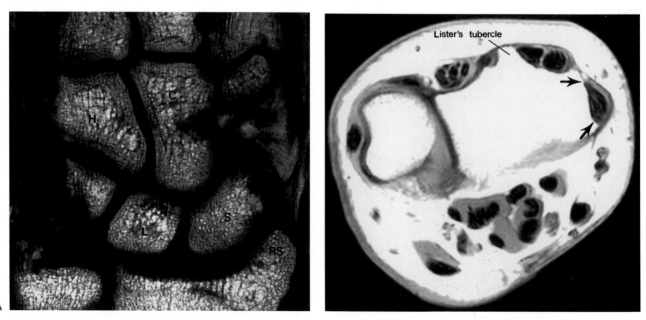

FIGURE 1-2. A: Coronal T1-weighted image demonstrating the radial styloid (RS), scaphoid (S), lunate (L), capitate (C), and hamate (H). **B:** Axial T1-weighted MR image demonstrating the lateral groove *(arrows)* for the extensor pollicis brevis and abductor pollicis longus tendons. Lister's tubercle is seen on the dorsal aspect of the radius.

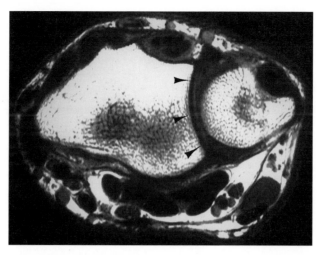

FIGURE 1-3. Axial T1-weighted MR image demonstrating the sigmoid notch *(arrowheads)* in the ulnar aspect of the radius.

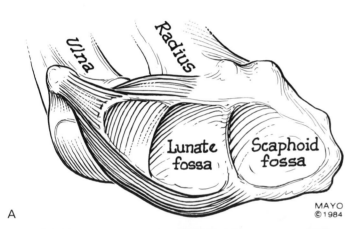

A

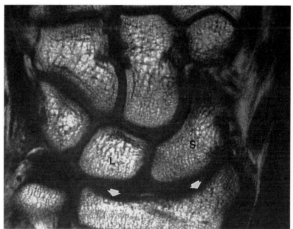

B

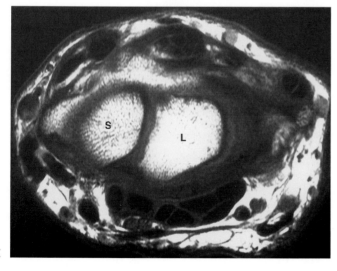

C

FIGURE 1-4. A: Illustration of the lunate and scaphoid fossae in the distal radius. (From Berquist TH. Imaging of orthopedic trauma. New York: Raven Press, 1992.) **B, C:** Coronal **(B)** and axial **(C)** T1-weighted images demonstrating the scaphoid (S) and lunate (L), and their position on the respective fossae *(arrows).*

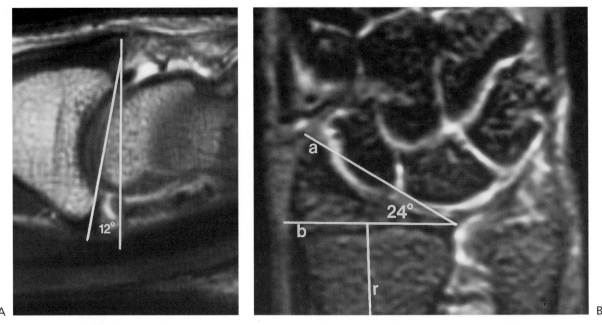

A   B

FIGURE 1-5. A: Sagittal MR arthrogram image demonstrating the normal 12° palmar tilt of the radial articular surface. **B:** Coronal MR image demonstrating the normal radial inclination angle of 24°. The angle is formed by a line from the styloid tip to the ulnar articular margin (a) and a line (b) perpendicular to the radial shaft (r) at the level of the ulnar articular margin.

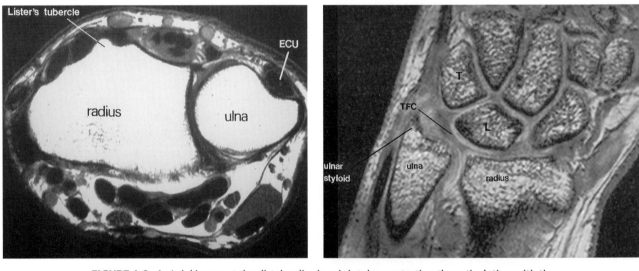

A   B

FIGURE 1-6. A: Axial image at the distal radioulnar joint demonstrating the articulation with the radius and dorsal ulnar notch for the sixth dorsal compartment and extensor carpi ulnaris (ECU) tendon. **B:** Coronal gradient echo image demonstrates the distal ulna and ulnar styloid, triangular fibrocartilage (TFC), and articulation with the lunate (L), triquetrum (T), and radius.

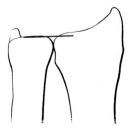

Neutral ulnar variance

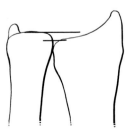

Positive ulnar variance

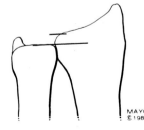

Negative ulnar variance

FIGURE 1-7. Illustration of neutral, positive (ulna longer than radial margin [line]), and negative (ulnar shorter than radial margin [line]) variance.

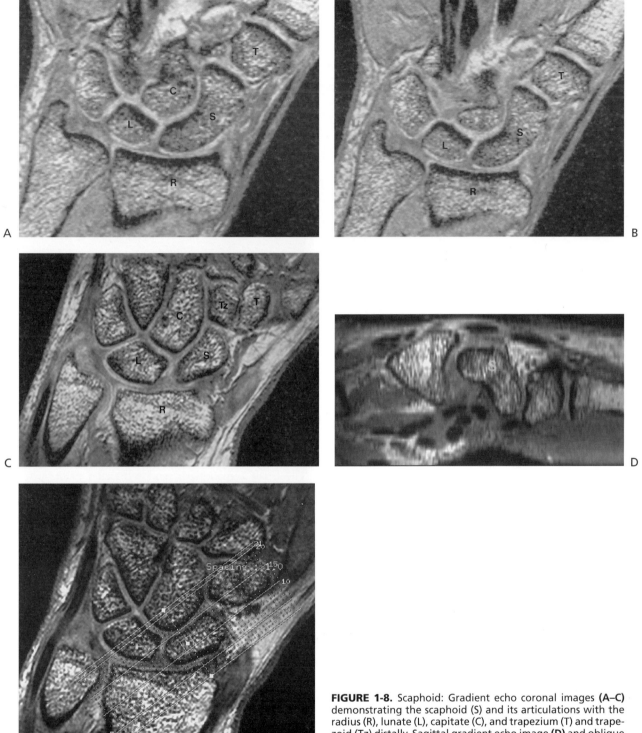

FIGURE 1-8. Scaphoid: Gradient echo coronal images **(A–C)** demonstrating the scaphoid (S) and its articulations with the radius (R), lunate (L), capitate (C), and trapezium (T) and trapezoid (Tz) distally. Sagittal gradient echo image **(D)** and oblique planes **(E)** required to demonstrate the scaphoid in the sagittal plane.

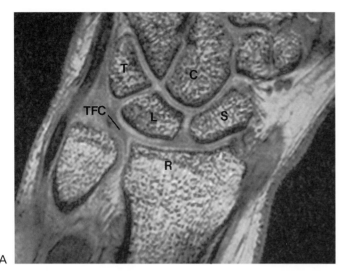

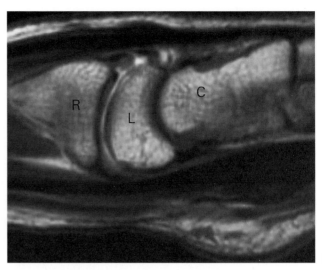

A   B

FIGURE 1-9. Lunate: **A:** Coronal gradient echo image demonstrating the lunate (L) and its articulations with the triangular fibrocartilage (TFC), radius (R), scaphoid (S), triquetrum (T), and capitate (C). This is type 1 lunate (no hamate articulation). **B:** Sagittal T1-weighted MR arthrogram demonstrating the moon-shaped appearance of the lunate (L) and aligned articulations with the radius (R) and capitate (C).

complex (Fig. 1-11). Type 1 is seen with ulnar minus variance. The lunate appears triangular or conical in the coronal plane. Type 2 configuration is rectangular and type 3, seen with ulnar positive variance, is linear on the distal articular surface and convex proximally.[31]

Triquetrum

The triquetrum is a well-vascularized structure with four articular facets (Fig. 1-12). The proximal convex surface articulates with the ulna and triangular fibrocartilage com-

plex. The distal concave surface articulates with the hamate. The radial surface articulates with the lunate. The distal anterior surface articulates with the pisiform. The anterior and posterior (dorsal) surfaces are roughened for ligament attachments.[16,35]

Pisiform

The flexor carpi ulnaris tendon attaches to the pisiform. Therefore, this carpal bone functions as a sesamoid bone (Fig. 1-13). Distal ligaments attach the pisiform to the hamate hook and fourth and fifth metacarpal bases.[35] The pisiform has one facet, which articulates with the triquetrum (Fig. 1-12).[11,35]

Trapezium

The trapezium has four articular surfaces. The ulnar facet articulates with the trapezoid, a concave proximal facet articulates with the scaphoid, and distally there is a small facet for articulating with the base of the second metacarpal and a larger facet for the first metacarpal (Fig. 1-14).[16,35]

On the volar or palmar aspect, there is a groove for the flexor carpi radialis tendon and a prominent ridge (trapezial ridge) for attachment of the flexor retinaculum and scaphotrapezial and anterior oblique ligaments (Fig. 1-14).[16]

Trapezoid

Like the trapezium, the trapezoid has four articular surfaces (Fig. 1-15).[9] The distal articular surface is wedge shaped for articulating with the second metacarpal. Approximately one third of patients have a small facet that articulates with the third metacarpal.[16] There are flat facets on the radial

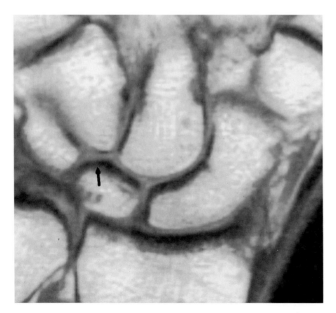

FIGURE 1-10. Coronal T1-weighted image demonstrating a type 2 lunate with a small *(arrow)* hamate facet.

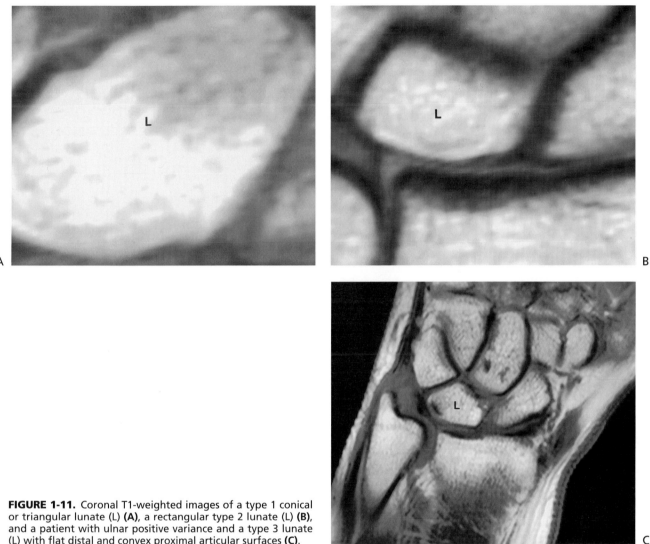

FIGURE 1-11. Coronal T1-weighted images of a type 1 conical or triangular lunate (L) **(A)**, a rectangular type 2 lunate (L) **(B)**, and a patient with ulnar positive variance and a type 3 lunate (L) with flat distal and convex proximal articular surfaces **(C)**.

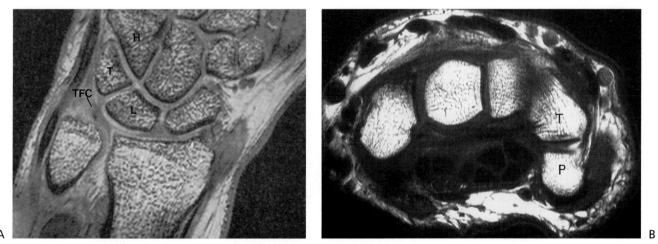

FIGURE 1-12. Triquetrum: **A:** Coronal gradient echo image demonstrating the articulations of the triquetrum (T) with the triangular fibrocartilage (TFC), lunate (L), and hamate (H). **B:** Axial T1-weighted image demonstrating articulation of the triquetrum (T) with the pisiform (P).

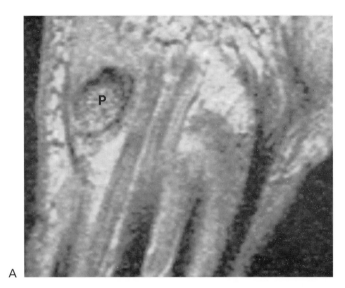

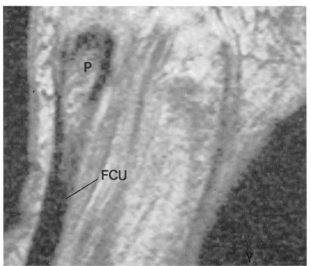

FIGURE 1-13. Coronal gradient echo images demonstrating the pisiform (P) in **(A)** and the flexor carpi ulnaris (FCU) tendon attaching to the pisiform (P) in **(B)**.

and ulnar aspect of the trapezoid for articulating with the trapezium and capitate.[9,16,35] The trapezoid articulates with the scaphoid proximally.

Capitate

The capitate is the largest carpal bone and plays an important role in the transverse carpal arch (Fig. 1-16).[17] The proximal capitate is termed the head of the capitate. The head is covered with articular cartilage with three surfaces that articulate with the scaphoid, lunate, and hamate.[35]

The distal radial aspect of the capitate is termed the body. The body of the capitate has a distal facet that articulates with the trapezoid. There are also distal facets that articulate with the third metacarpal and a smaller facet for the second metacarpal.[16,35] In about 85% of patients, there is a small facet for the fourth metacarpal base (Fig. 1-16).[45]

Hamate

The hamate has a prominent palmar projection (the hook), which forms the medial boundary of the carpal tunnel (Fig. 1-16A). The tip of the hook serves for attachment of the flexor retinaculum, pisohamatum ligament, and opponens digiti minimi muscle.[16,35]

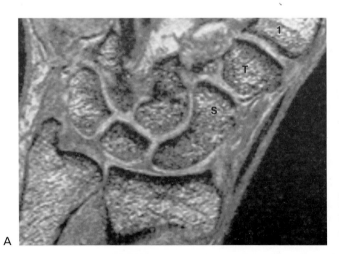

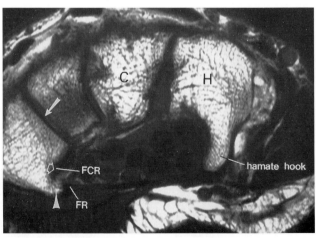

FIGURE 1-14. Trapezium: **A:** Coronal gradient echo image demonstrating the concave articulation of the trapezium (T) with the scaphoid (S) and the first metacarpal base (1). **B:** Axial T1-weighted image of the distal carpal row demonstrating the trapezium and its articulation with the trapezoid *(arrow)*. There is a groove *(open arrow)* for the flexor carpi radialis (FCR) tendon and a ridge *(arrowhead)* for attachment of the flexor retinaculum (FR) and volar ligaments. C, capitate; H, hamate.

FIGURE 1-15. Trapezoid: **A:** Axial T1-weighted image demonstrating the articulations of the trapezoid (Tz) with the trapezium (T) and capitate (C). **B, C:** Coronal gradient echo images demonstrating the articulation with the scaphoid (S) **(B)** and the wedge-shaped articulation **(C)** with the base of the second metacarpal (2).

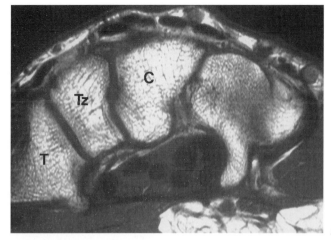

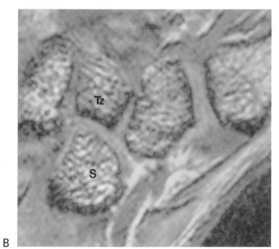

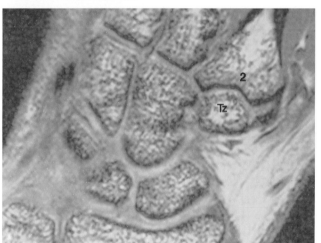

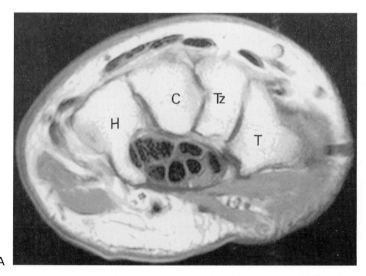

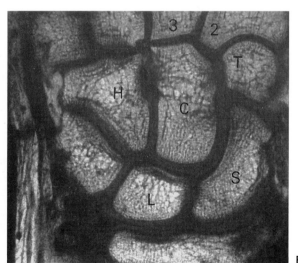

FIGURE 1-16. Capitate and hamate. Axial **(A)** and coronal **(B)** T1-weighted images demonstrating the capitate (C) and its articulations with the hamate (H), trapezoid (Tz), lunate (L), scaphoid (S), trapezium (T), and second (2) and third (3) metatarsal bases distally.

Distally, the hamate articulates with the fourth and fifth metacarpal bases. There is an articular facet proximally and medially for the triquetrum. The radial aspect articulates with the capitate (Fig. 1-16B).[9,35]

Metacarpals and Phalanges

The proximal metacarpals articulate with the distal carpal row (Fig. 1-1). There is little motion at these joints except at the first carpometacarpal articulation.[9,35]

The proximal and middle phalanges are similar in structure with proximal and distal flaring. These structures are primarily canallous bone.[9] The thumb lacks a middle phalanx and has two phalanges. The remaining digits have three phalanges (Fig. 1-1).[4,9,35]

ARTICULAR AND LIGAMENT ANATOMY

Wrist

The wrist is composed of six articulations: (1) distal radioulnar joint, (2) radiocarpal, (3) midcarpal, (4) pisotriquetral, (5) trapeziometacarpal, and (6) common carpometacarpal joints (Fig. 1-17).[9,35]

Nontraumatic communications may occur between the distal radioulnar and radiocarpal joints in 7% of patients in the third decade and 53% during the seventh decade.[28] In addition, communications between the midcarpal and radiocarpal joints may be noted in 43% of scapholunate and 55% of lunotriquetral articulations in patients older than 40 years.[29] The pisotriquetral joint communicates with the pretriquetralis recess of the radiocarpal joint in 30% of patients.[29]

Distal Radioulnar Joint

The distal radioulnar joint is stabilized primarily by the triangular fibrocartilage complex (TFCC) (Fig. 1-18).[9] The articular disc is composed of fibrocartilage and has a similar appearance to the meniscus of the knee on MR images.[10] The disc attaches to the ulnar margin of the distal radius at the distal margin of the sigmoid notch. The broader ulnar portion of the TFCC attaches to the ulnar styloid, the adjacent ulna fovea, and the deep lamina of the antebrachial fascia.[16,31] The deep lamina is separated from the superficial lamina by the extensor carpi ulnaris tendon and its sheath (Fig. 1-18).[16]

The ulnar portion of the TFCC is vascularized by branches of the ulnar and posterior interosseous arteries. The central and radial aspects are essentially avascular.[16] The central region frequently degenerates after age 40 resulting in signal abnormalities (increased signal intensity) on MR images (Fig. 1-19).[11,41]

The remainder of the TFCC consists of the dorsal and palmar distal radioulnar ligaments, and the ulnar collateral

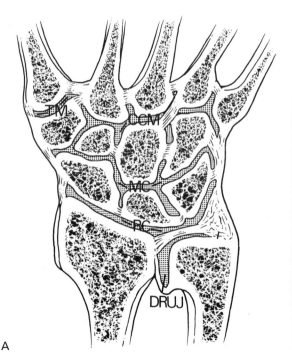

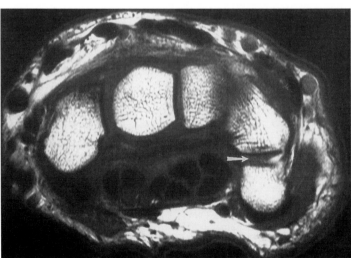

A   B

FIGURE 1-17. A: Coronal illustration of the distal radioulnar joint (DRUJ), radiocarpal (RC), midcarpal (MC), common carpometacarpal (CCM), and trapeziometacarpal (TM) joints. The pisotriquetral joint is only seen in the axial or sagittal planes. Axial T1-weighted image **(B)** demonstrates the pisotriquetral articulation *(arrow)*.

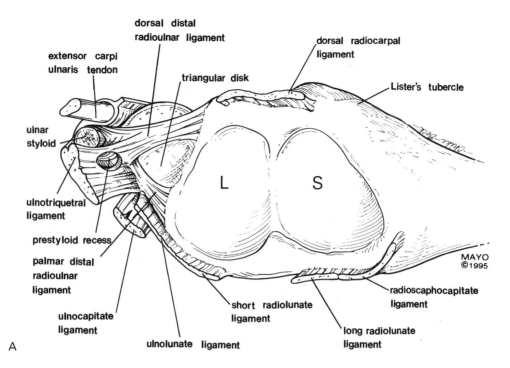

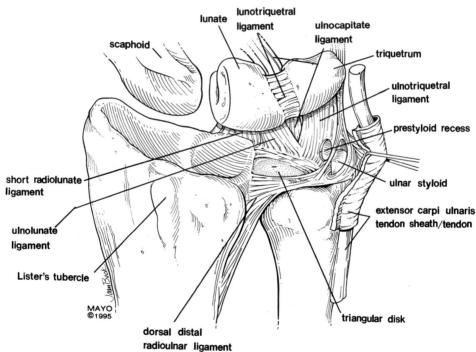

FIGURE 1-18. A: Illustration of the distal radius (L, lunate fossa; S, scaphoid fossa), ligament attachments, and triangular fibrocartilage complex with radioulnar ligaments. **B:** Illustration of the ulnocarpal ligament complex and triangular fibrocartilage complex seen from the dorsal aspect. Note the relationship of the prestyloid recess and the ulnotriquetral ligaments. (From Berger RA. Ligament anatomy. In: Cooney WP III, Linscheid RL, Dobyns JH, eds. The wrist: diagnosis and operative treatment. St. Louis: Mosby, 1998:73–105.)

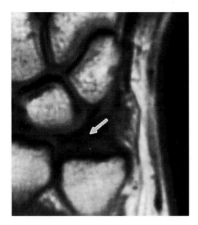

FIGURE 1-19. Coronal T1-weighted image of the triangular fibrocartilage demonstrating increased signal intensity *(arrow)* due to disc degeneration.

ligament. The triangular fibrocartilage is composed of the disc and radioulnar ligaments (Fig. 1-18).[2,34]

Radiocarpal Joint and Ligaments

The radiocarpal ligaments are divided into palmar and dorsal groups.[5–7] The palmar radiocarpal ligaments attach 1 to 2 mm proximal to the radial articular surface and, except for the radioscaphocapitate ligament, all attach to the osseous structures of the proximal carpal row (Fig. 1-20).[5]

Palmar Ligaments

Radioscaphocapitate ligament (Fig. 1-20A). The most lateral of the palmar ligaments originates at the radial styloid and palmar radial margin and extends obliquely to the scaphoid waist and then to the capitate where it joins the ulnocapitate ligament to form the arcuate ligament.[5,7,35]

Long radiolunate ligament (Fig. 1-20A). The long radiolunate ligament takes its origin from the palmar distal radius medial to the radioscaphocapitate ligament. The ligament overlaps the radioscaphocapitate ligament as it courses obliquely to insert on the palmar radial aspect of the lunate.[5,7,13]

Radioscapholunate ligament (ligament of Testut) (Fig. 1-20A). The radioscapholunate ligament originates on the ulnar aspect of the distal radius. The ligament has a vertical orientation as it originates from the palmar capsule and extends between the long and short radiolunate ligaments to insert on the lunate and medial scaphoid.[5,13]

Short radiolunate ligament (Figs. 1-20A and 1-21). The short radiolunate ligament originates at the palmar medial radius and extends distally as a wide band that forms the

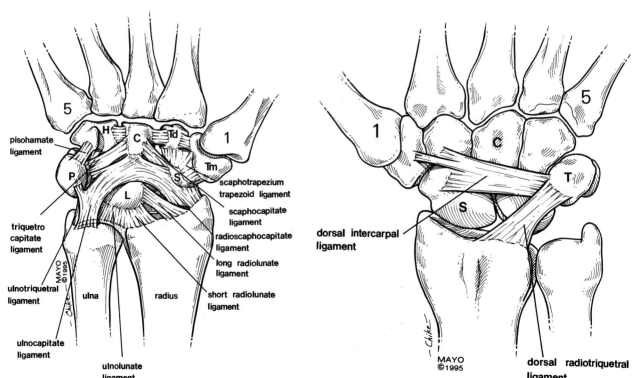

FIGURE 1-20. Illustrations of the palmar **(A)** and dorsal **(B)** carpal ligaments. Captions: 1, first metacarpal; 5, fifth metacarpal; Tm, trapezium; Td, trapezoid; C, capitate; H, hamate; P, pisiform; L, lunate; S, scaphoid; T, triquetrum. (From Berger RA. Ligament anatomy. In: Cooney WP III, Linscheid RL, Dobyns JH, eds. The wrist: diagnosis and operative treatment. St. Louis: Mosby, 1998:73–105.)

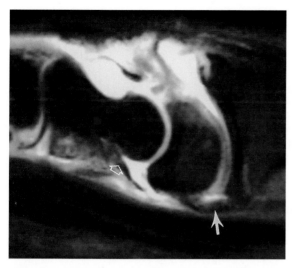

FIGURE 1-21. Sagittal MR arthrogram image demonstrating the short radiolunate *(arrow)* and junction of the radioscaphocapitate and ulnocapitate ligaments as they attach to the palmar surface of the capitate *(open arrow)*.

floor of the radiolunate space before inserting on the palmar surface of the lunate.[5,7,13]

Dorsal Ligaments

Dorsal radiocarpal ligament (Fig. 1-20B). The dorsal radiocarpal ligament takes its broad origin from the distal radius on the ulnar side of Lister's tubercle. The ligament has an oblique ulnar course to insert on the triquetrum (superficial fibers) and lunate (deep fibers). This ligament forms the floor of the fourth-sixth-extensor tendon compartments.[5,7,13]

Dorsal intercarpal ligament (Figs. 1-20B and 1-22). The dorsal intercarpal ligament takes its origin from the tri-

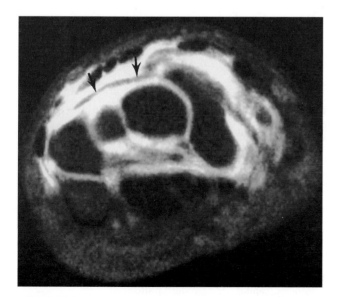

FIGURE 1-22. Axial MR arthrogram demonstrating the dorsal ligaments *(arrows)*.

quetrum and extends transversely to insert by three slips on the scaphoid, trapezium, and trapezoid.[5,13]

Ulnocarpal Ligaments

The ulnocarpal ligaments originate primarily from the palmar radioulnar ligament at the margin of the triangular fibrocartilage complex (Fig. 1-18).[5,35]

Ulnolunate ligament (Fig. 1-18). The ulnolunate ligament is contiguous with the short radiolunate ligament. The two ligaments blend together such that only the origin (palmar radioulnar ligament) separates it from the short radiolunate ligament.[5,13]

Ulnotriquetral ligament (Fig. 1-18) The ulnotriquetral ligament takes its origin just medial to the ulnolunate from the palmar radioulnar ligament. As described by Berger,[5] this ligament is complex with fibers coursing distally to insert on the triquetrum. This is not consistent due to the pisotriquetral orifice seen in 70% of adults. The orifice forms in communication between the radiocarpal and pisotriquetral joints on MR arthrograms. The main portion of the ulnotriquetral ligament is medial to this orifice and inserts on the medial triquetral margin.[5,13] The prestyloid recess is consistently present in the ulnotriquetral ligament and inconsistently communicates with the ulnar styloid (Fig. 1-23).[5]

Ulnocapitate ligament (Fig. 1-20). The ulnocapitate ligament originates from the base of the ulnar styloid and palmar radioulnar ligament. It takes a course palmar to the above ulnocarpal ligaments and inserts on the triquetrum, pisiform and pisotriquetral ligament before blending with the radioscaphocapitate ligament with its capitate insertion to form the ulnar side of the arcuate ligament.[5,13]

Palmar Midcarpal Ligaments

The palmar midcarpal ligaments are contiguous with the radiocarpal and ulnar carpal ligaments as they join to form a nearly contiguous palmar capsule volar to the intercarpal joints.[5,35]

Scaphotrapezium trapezoid ligament (Fig. 1-24). The scaphotrapezium trapezoid ligament takes its origin from the distal palmar scaphoid. As the ligament courses distally it forms two bands; one attaching to the trapezium and the second inserting on the trapezoid.[5]

Scaphocapitate ligament (Fig. 1-24). The scaphocapitate ligament is distal to the radioscaphocapitate ligament as it takes an oblique course from the distal medial scaphoid to the radial aspect of the body of the capitate.[5,13,35]

Triquetrocapitate ligament (Fig. 1-24). The triquetrocapitate ligament courses obliquely and just distal to the ulnocapitate ligament as it takes an oblique course from the triquetrum to the ulnar aspect of the body of the capitate.[5,13]

Triquetrohamate ligament (Fig. 1-24). The triquetrohamate ligament takes its origin from the palmar radial surface

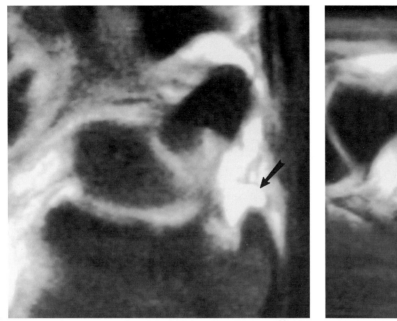 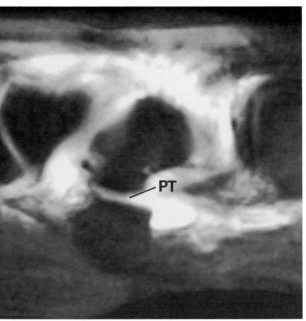

FIGURE 1-23. Coronal **(A)** and sagittal **(B)** MR arthrogram images demonstrating the prestyloid recess *(arrow)*. The pisotriquetral (PT) joint is seen in **(B)**.

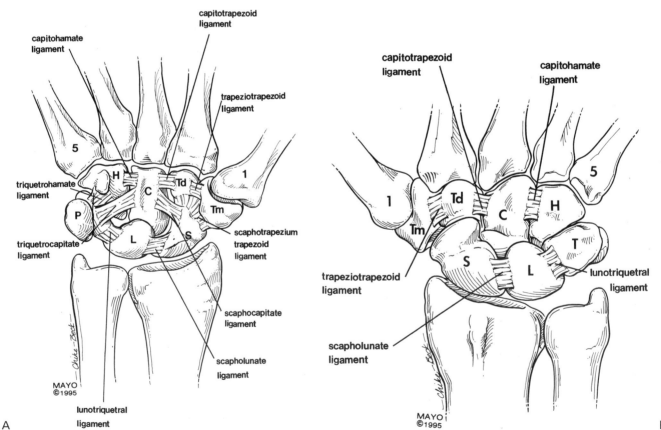

FIGURE 1-24. Illustration of the palmar **(A)** and dorsal **(B)** intercarpal ligaments; C, capitate; H, hamate; L, lunate; P, pisiform; S, scaphoid; Td, trapezoid; Tm, trapezium; 1, first metacarpal; 5, fifth metacarpal. (From Berger RA. Ligament anatomy. In: Cooney WP III, Linscheid RL, Dobyns JH, eds. The wrist: diagnosis and operative treatment. St. Louis: Mosby, 1998:73–105.)

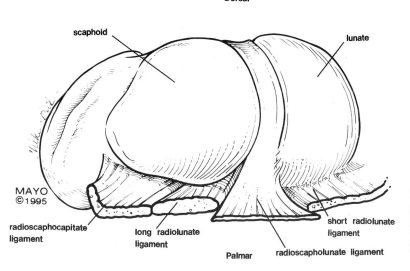

FIGURE 1-25. Illustration of the scapholunate complex from proximally and slightly radial perspective. (From Berger RA. Ligament anatomy. In: Cooney WP III, Linscheid RL, Dobyns JH, eds. The wrist: diagnosis and operative treatment. St. Louis: Mosby, 1998:73–105.)

of the triquetrum distal to the triquetrocapitate ligament. This broad ligament courses obliquely to insert on the hamate at the margin of the hamate hook.[5]

Pisohamate ligament (Fig. 1-24). The pisohamate ligament is a continuation of the flexor carpi ulnaris tendon distal to the pisiform. This ligament is the floor of Guyon's canal with a short course to insert on the top of the hamate hook.[5]

Interosseous Ligaments

The scapholunate and lunotriquetral ligaments are "C" shaped so the distal articular surfaces communicate with the intercarpal (midcarpal) joint (Fig. 1-25). The ligaments extend from the dorsal to the proximal and palmar aspects of the joint surfaces.[5] The scapholunate ligament is thicker dorsally than the proximal or palmar portions.[5,8] Both the dorsal and palmar positions of the lunotriquetral ligament are thicker than the proximal portion;[5,37] therefore, the appearance of the ligament varies on MR images depending on the plane of section (Fig. 1-26).[5,9,11,37,39,40]

The pisotriquetral ligament may completely encapsulate the articular surface or have a U-shaped configuration on those patients where the pisotriquetral joint communicates with the radiocarpal joint.[5,39]

The trapezium-trapezoid interosseous ligament, unlike those ligaments described in the proximal row, consist of transverse dorsal and palmar bands with no deep interosseous component.[5,13,35]

The trapeziocapitate and capitohamate ligaments have dorsal and palmar components but also deep interosseous ligaments between the articulating surfaces (Figs. 1-27 and 1-28).[5]

Ligamentous anatomy of the metacarpophalangeal (Fig. 1-29) and interphalangeal joints (Fig. 1-30) is similar with collateral ligaments and volar ligaments closely incorporated

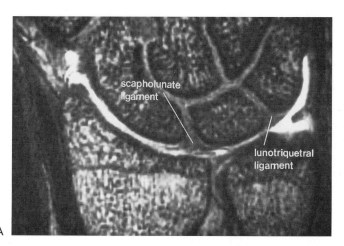

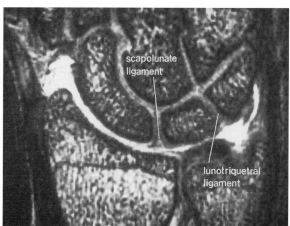

FIGURE 1-26. Coronal gradient echo MR arthrogram images **(A, B)** at different levels demonstrating variation in thickness of the scapholunate and lunotriquetral ligaments.

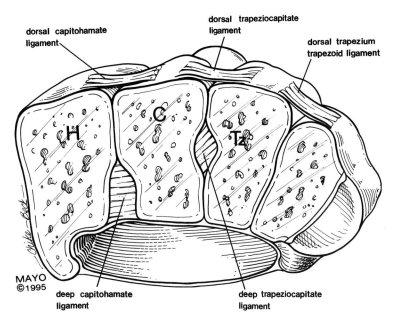

FIGURE 1-27. Illustration of dorsal and interosseous components of the distal carpal row. H-hamate, C-capitate, Tz-trapezoid. (From Berger RA. Ligament Anatomy. In Cooney WP III, Linscheid RL, Dobyns JH, eds. The wrist: diagnosis and operative treatment. St. Louis: Mosby, 1998:73–105.)

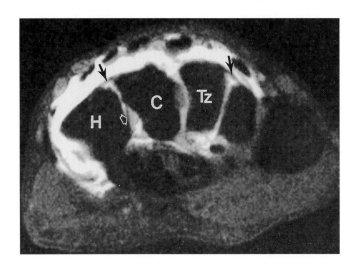

FIGURE 1-28. Axial MR arthrogram image demonstrating the dorsal *(arrows)* and interosseous *(open arrow)* ligaments of the distal carpal row. H, hamate; C, capitate; Tz, trapezoid.

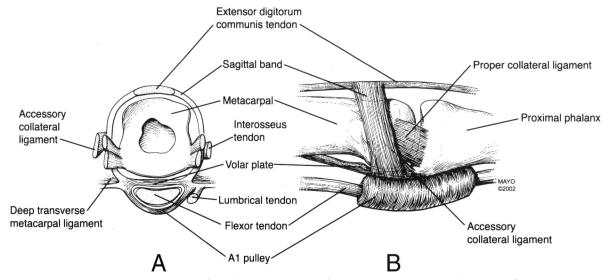

FIGURE 1-29. Illustration of the ligament support of the metacarpophalangeal joint seen from the **(A)** axial and lateral **(B)** projections.

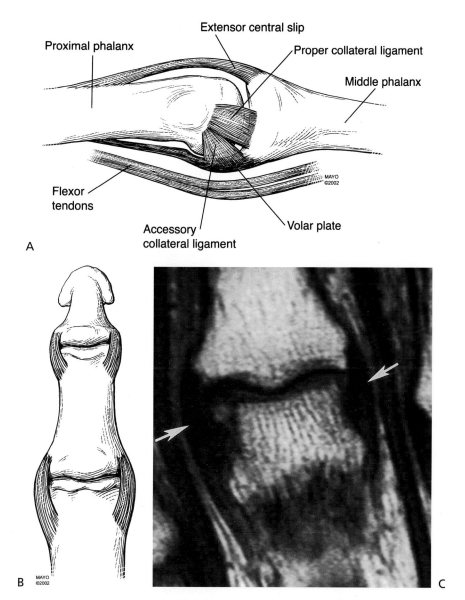

Proximal phalanx

Extensor central slip

Proper collateral ligament

Middle phalanx

Flexor tendons

Accessory collateral ligament

Volar plate

A

B

C

FIGURE 1-30. Illustrations of the interphalangeal anatomy of the proximal interphalangeal (PIP) joint **(A)** and collateral ligaments of the PIP and distal interphalangeal (DIP) joints seen in the coronal plane **(B)**. Coronal T1-weighted MR image **(C)** demonstrating the collateral ligaments *(arrows)* at the PIP joint.

with the joint capsule (Figs. 1-29 to 1-32).[9,11,41] The collateral ligaments are seen in the axial and coronal planes (Figs. 1-31 and 1-32) on MR images. The ligaments blend with the capsule on the radial and ulnar side of the joint.[41] These ligaments are tight in extension and relax in flexion.[9,11] The palmar plate is clearly visible on sagittal (Fig. 1-31) and axial MR images.[41]

MUSCULAR ANATOMY

Many muscles and tendons that cross the wrist originate at the elbow or proximal forearm. The muscles of the forearm are largely responsible for flexion and extension of the wrist (Fig. 1-33). This section primarily deals with muscles directly related to bones of the hand and wrist with regard to their origins and insertions (Table 1-1).[12,22,23]

The chief flexors of the wrist are the flexor carpi radialis and flexor carpi ulnaris. The palmaris longus is a minor flexor of the wrist. Extension of the wrist is largely due to the extensor carpi radialis longus and brevis and the extensor carpi ulnaris. During radial deviation of the wrist, the primary muscles involved are the abductor pollicis longus and the extensor pollicis brevis. Ulnar deviation of the wrist is accomplished primarily by the extensor carpi ulnaris.[12,35]

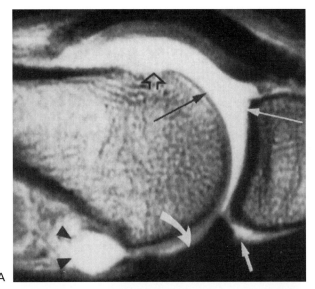

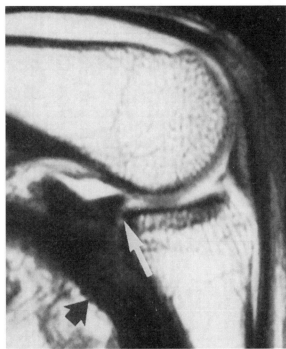

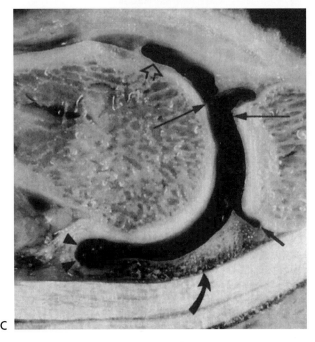

FIGURE 1-31. T1-weighted arthrogram images of the third metacarpophalangeal (MCP) joint in extension **(A)** and flexion **(B)**, anatomic section in extension **(C)**. The palmar plate *(curved arrow)* and distal recess *(short arrow)* and the loose proximal recess *(arrowheads)* are shown in **(A)** and **(C)**. A bare area *(open arrow)* is seen between the cartilage *(long straight arrow)* and the dorsal capsule insertion in **(A)** and **(C)**. The palmar plate angles and the distal recess *(white arrow)* compresses in flexion **(B)**. The flexor tendon *(black arrow* in **(B))** is adjacent to bone. (From Theumann NH, Pfirrmann CWA, Trudell DJ, et al. MR imaging of the metacarpophalangeal joint of the fingers. Conventional MR imaging and MR arthrographic findings in cadavers. Radiology 2002;222:431–445.)

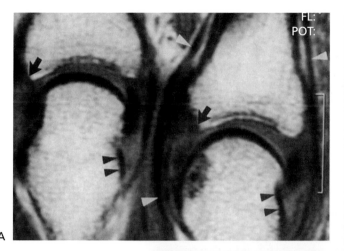

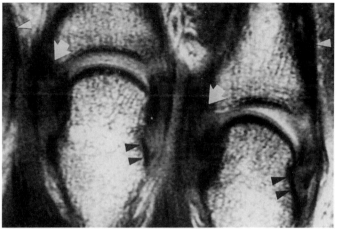

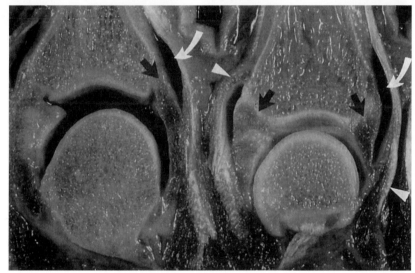

FIGURE 1-32. Coronal T1-weighted images **(A, B)** and anatomic section **(C)** of the second and third metacarpophalangeal (MCP) joints. *Black arrowheads* mark the proximal and *straight arrows* the distal ligament attachments in **(A, B).** Interosseous tendons *(white arrowheads)* are easily seen. There are spaces *(curved arrows)* between the ligaments and tendons **(C).** (From Theumann NH, Pfirrmann CWA, Trudell DJ, et al. MR imaging of the metacarpophalangeal joint of the fingers. Conventional MR imaging and MR arthrographic findings in cadavers. Radiology 2002;222:431–445.)

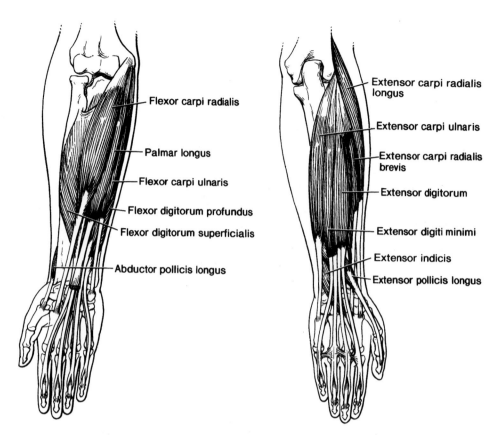

FIGURE 1-33. Illustration of the flexor and extensor muscle groups.

TABLE 1-1. MUSCLES OF THE HAND

Muscle	Origin	Insertion Site	Action	Innervation Site
Lumbricals (4)	Tendons of flexor digitorum profundus	Extensor aponeurosis	Extensors of interphalangeal joints	Radial or 1st and 2nd lumbricals–medium nerve, 3rd and 4th ulnar nerve
Flexor pollicis longus	Anterior middle one-third radius and interosseous membrane	Distal phalanx thumb	Flexor of thumb	Median nerve (anterior interosseous branch)
Interossei				
Palmar (3)	2nd, 4th, 5th metacarpal diaphysis	Extensor aponeurosis, proximal phalanges	Abduction and adduction of fingers	Deep branch of ulnar nerve
Dorsal (4)	1st to 5th metacarpal diaphyses			
Abductor pollicis brevis	Flexor retinaculum, trapezium	Radial side proximal, phalanx thumb	Abductor of thumb	Median nerve
Flexor pollicis brevis	Flexor retinaculum, trapezium, and trapezoid	Radial flexor aspect, proximal phalanx, thumb	Flexes and rotates thumb	Median nerve
Opponens pollicis	Flexor retinaculum, trapezium	Radial diaphysis 1st metacarpal	Stabilize and opposition of thumb	Median nerve
Adductor pollicis	3rd metacarpal, trapezium, trapezoid, capitate	Base proximal phalanx, thumb		Median nerve
Palmaris brevis	Palmar aponeurosis (ulnar side)	Medial skin palm	Draws skin laterally	Deep branch ulnar nerve
Abductor digiti minimi	Pisiform	Ulnar base 5th proximal phalanx	Abductor 5th finger	Deep branch ulnar nerve
Flexor digiti minimi brevis	Hamate hook, flexor retinaculum	Ulnar base 5th proximal phalanx	Flexor 5th MCP joint	Deep branch ulnar nerve
Opponens digiti minimi	Flexor retinaculum, distal hamate hook	5th metacarpal diaphysis	Draws 5th metacarpal anteriorly	Deep branch ulnar nerve

Adapted from Berquist TH. *MRI of the musculoskeletal system,* 3rd ed. New York: Raven Press, 1996; Boles CA, Kannam S, Cardwell AB. The forearm: anatomy of muscle compartments and nerves. *AJR AM J Roentgenol* 2000;174:151–159; and Rosse C, Rosse PC. Hollingheads textbook of anatomy. Philadelphia: Lippincott–Raven Publishers, 1997, with permission.

Typically, four lumbrical muscles arise from the flexor digitorum profundus tendons and extend along the radial aspects of the second through fifth metacarpals to insert in the extensor aponeurosis of the proximal phalanx on the radial side (Fig. 1-34).[33] The muscles can be identified on MR images in the axial and coronal planes and are seen as tissue of muscle signal intensity between the flexor digitorum profundus tendons proximally and along the radial aspect of the metacarpals adjacent to the interosseous muscles more distally (Fig. 1-34).[11,35] Insertions are not usually clearly defined on MR images. The flexor pollicis longus is important in the hand and wrist. As noted in Table 1-1, the muscle originates from the anterior aspect of the middle third of the radius. The tendon passes through the radial side of the carpal tunnel radial to the superficial and deep flexor tendons. A synovial sheath of the flexor pollicis longus tendon (Figs. 1-34 and 1-35) begins just proximal to the flexor retinaculum and extends distally to near the insertion of the tendon on the distal phalanx of the thumb (Table 1-1).[11,35]

The interosseous muscles form the deepest layer of the muscles in the hand and are divided into palmar and dorsal groups (Fig. 1-34). The palmar group consists of three muscles that take their origin on the radial aspect of the fifth and fourth metacarpals and the ulnar aspect of the second metacarpal. The muscles pass distally between the metacarpophalangeal joints to insert on the extensor aponeurosis. The dorsal interossei originate from adjacent metacarpals, the first from the first and second metacarpal, the second from the second and third, the third from the third and fourth, and the fourth from the fourth and fifth metacarpal diaphyses. The muscles pass dorsally and distally to insert with a palmar and dorsal slip into the bases of the proximal phalanges. The interosseous muscles, both palmar and dorsal, are innervated by the deep branch of the ulnar nerve and function in abduction and adduction of the fingers of the hand (Table 1-1).[11,35]

The thenar eminence or muscle group (Fig. 1-34) comprises the abductor pollicis brevis and superficial head of the flexor pollicis brevis that overlie the opponens pollicis. The abductor pollicis brevis arises from the flexor retinaculum and has deeper origins from the trapezium and trapezoid. This triangular muscle extends distally to insert in the radial aspect of the proximal phalanx of the thumb. It serves as the primary abductor of the thumb. The flexor pollicis brevis has two heads, one superficial and the other deep. The superficial head arises from the trapezium and flexor retinaculum and the deep head from the trapezoid. The muscle extends distally to form a tendon that inserts on the radial flexor side of the base of the proximal phalanx of the thumb. The primary function is flexion and rotation of thumb. The opponens pollicis is partially covered by the abductors and flexors of the thumb and arises from the flexor retinaculum and trapezium to insert on the radial surface of the diaphysis of the first metacarpal. The adductor pollicis arises with both oblique and transverse heads. The transverse head arises from the ulnar surface of the third metacarpal diaphysis and the oblique head from the base of the third metacarpal and flexor aspects of the trapezium, trapezoid, and capitate. The triangular muscle extends to insert at the base of the proximal phalanx of the thumb. This muscle serves to adduct the metacarpal and flex the metacarpophalangeal joint of the thumb (Table 1-1).[11,35]

The hypothenar muscle group (Fig. 1-34) consists of one superficial and three deep muscles. The superficial muscle is the palmaris brevis that arises from the ulnar side of the palmar aponeurosis and extends medially to attach into the skin along the medial border of the palm. This muscle is superficial to the ulnar nerve and artery.[35] The deep muscles include the abductor digiti minimi, flexor digiti minimi brevis, and opponens digiti minimi. The abductor digiti minimi is the most superficial of the three deep muscles. It arises from the distal surface of the pisiform and passes distally along the medial aspect of the hand to insert along the ulnar side of the base of the fifth proximal phalanx. This muscle abducts the little finger at the metacarpophalangeal joint. It acts along with the dorsal interosseous muscle to assist in abduction or spreading of the fingers. The flexor digiti minimi brevis arises more distally than the abductor digiti minimi and takes its origin from the hook of the hamate and flexor retinaculum. This muscle passes more obliquely and medially and inserts in the same position as the abductor. The main function of this muscle is a flexor of the fifth metacarpophalangeal joint. The third and final muscle of the deep hypothenar group is the opponens digiti minimi. This muscle is the deepest and arises deep to the abductor and flexor from the flexor retinaculum and distal hook of the hamate, taking an oblique course to insert along the ulnar aspect of the fifth metacarpal diaphysis. This muscle draws the fifth metacarpal anteriorly. All muscles of the hypothenar group are supplied by the deep branch of the ulnar nerve (Table 1-1).[11,35]

Numerous muscular variations have been described. The muscular anomalies and variants will be discussed in Chapter 3.

TENDON ANATOMY

Knowledge of the flexor and extensor tendon mechanisms and tendon sheath locations is important for image technique selection and to provide the necessary road maps for surgical repair.[1,9,20,24,34]

Flexor Tendons

The flexor tendons begin in the distal third of the forearm.[9,11,35] For purposes of function and repair, the tendons are divided into five zones for the hand and wrist and two zones for the thumb (Fig. 1-35).[43] There are multiple variations, but in general, as the flexor pollicis longus

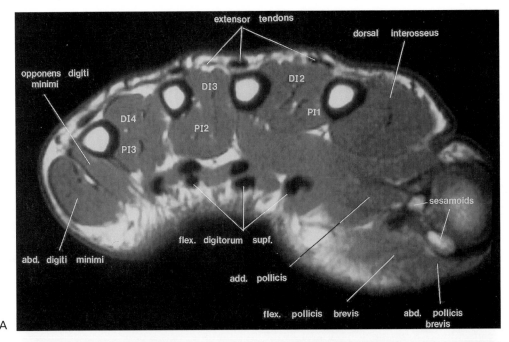

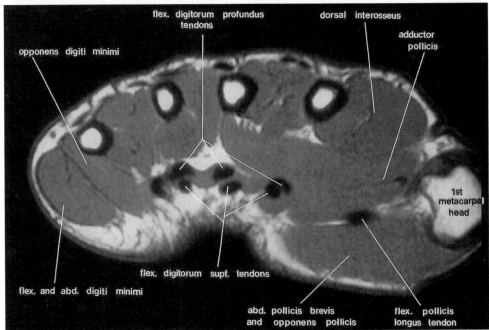

FIGURE 1-34. Axial MR images at the level of the metacarpal bases **(A)**, first metacarpal head **(B)**, and mid-metacarpals **(C)**, and coronal **(D, E)** images demonstrating the muscles of the hand. DI, dorsal interosseous; PI, palmar interosseous.

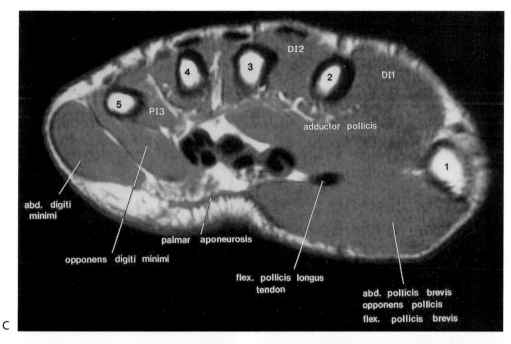

C

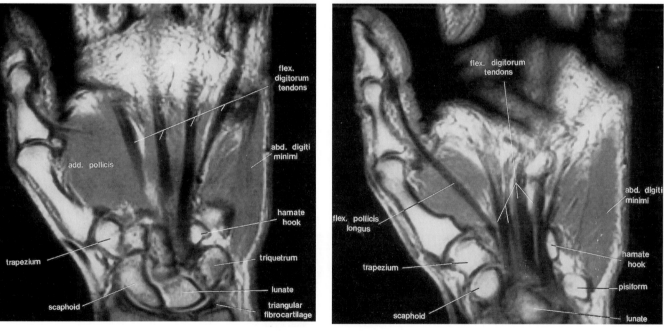

D

E

FIGURE 1-34. (*continued*)

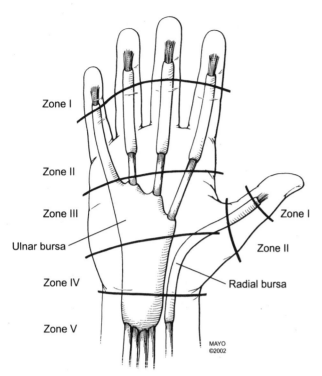

FIGURE 1-35. Illustration of the flexor tendons, their sheaths and anatomic zones.

(FPL) tendon passes the transverse flexor retinaculum it enters a continuous sheath that becomes the radial bursa (Fig. 1-35).[19,35] The FPL tendon is dorsal and radial to the median nerve as it passes through the carpal tunnel to insert on the distal phalanx of the thumb (Fig. 1-35).[11,15,35]

The flexor digitorum superficialis and profundus tendons lie dorsal and medial to the median nerve in the carpal tunnel and are enclosed in a common sheath (ulnar bursa) to the distal margin of the flexor retinaculum.[1,35] At this point the sheath continues along the tendon for the 5th finger but the index, middle, and ring fingers have separate tendon sheaths that begin at the level of the metacarpal necks (Figs. 1-35 and 1-36).[42]

The flexor carpi radialis tendon courses along the radial aspect of the carpal tunnel and is separated from the other tendons by the deep lamina of the flexor retinaculum.[1,4] This tendon can be seen on axial images in a shallow groove in the ulnar margin of the trapezium prior to insertion on base of the second metacarpal.[1]

The flexor carpi ulnaris tendon is superficial and inserts on the pisiform with fibers continuing distally to form the ligamentous attachment to the hamate hook and fourth and fifth metacarpal bases.[1,5]

Distal to the metacarpal phalangeal joints there are five annular and three C-shaped pulleys that are thickened areas in the tendon sheath (Fig. 1-37).[20,42] The annular pulleys prevent bowstringing with flexion. The C pulleys allow the sheath to conform to position with flexion.[43] Annular bands A2 and A4 (Fig. 1-37) are most important. Similarly, there are three pulleys for the thumb.[20,43]

Extensor Tendons

The extensor mechanism arises from multiple muscle bellies in the forearm. The extensor tendons are stabilized by the extensor retinaculum with septations dividing the extensor tendons into six compartments (Fig. 1-38).[1,11,23,35] The first dorsal compartment is located along the lateral margin of the distal radius and contains the abductor pollicis longus and extensor pollicis brevis tendons.[1,11,35] The second dorsal compartment is located lateral to Lister's tubercle

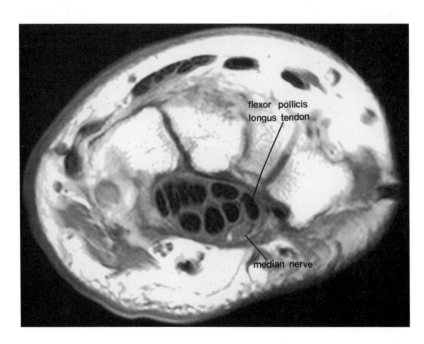

FIGURE 1-36. Axial MR image demonstrating the relationship of the flexor pollicis longus to the median nerve.

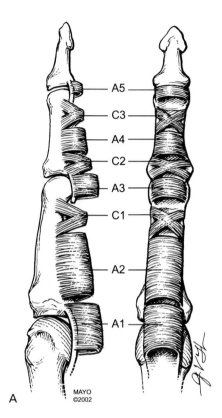

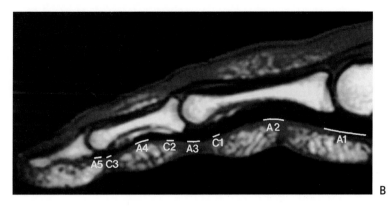

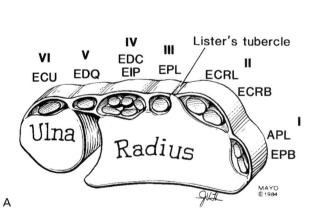

FIGURE 1-37. A: Illustration of the retinacular sheath of the flexor tendons. **B:** Sagittal MR image with pulley locations marked.

and contains the extensor carpi radialis longus and brevis tendons.[4,11,35] The third compartment is on the ulnar side of Lister's tubercle and contains the extensor pollicis longus tendon. The fourth compartment lies over the dorsal medial radius and contains the extensor digitorum and extensor indicis proprius tendons. The fifth compartment overlies the radioulnar joint and contains the extensor digiti quinti (minimi) tendon. The sixth compartment lies in a dorsal ulnar groove and contains the extensor carpi ulnaris tendon (Fig. 1-38).[1,11,35]

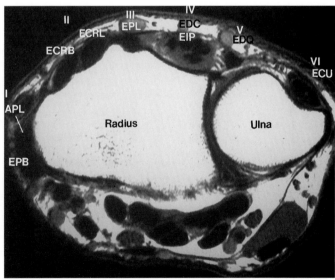

FIGURE 1-38. A: Cross-sectional illustration of the extensor tendon compartments of the wrist. **B:** Corresponding axial MR image. ECU, extensor carpi ulnaris; EDQ, extensor digiti quinti proprius; EDC, extensor digitorum communis; EIP, extensor indicus proprius; EPL, extensor pollicis longus; ECRL, extensor carpi radialis longus; ECRB, extensor carpi radialis brevis; APL, abductor pollicis longus; EPB, extensor pollicis brevis.

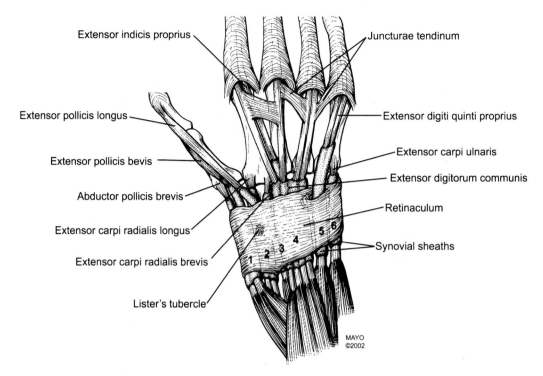

FIGURE 1-39. Illustration of extensor retinaculum, tendon sheaths, and tendons. Compartments are numbered 1 through 6.

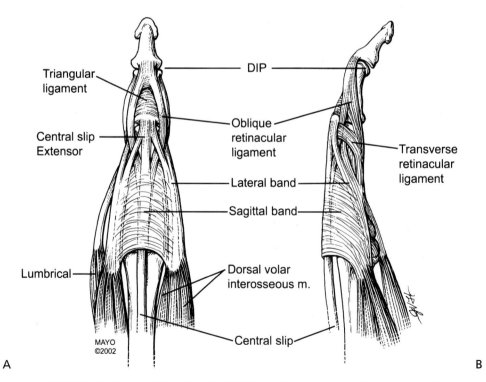

FIGURE 1-40. Coronal **(A)** and sagittal **(B)** illustrations of extensor tendon support.

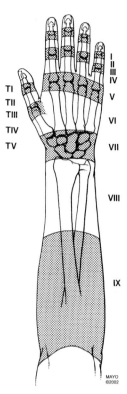

FIGURE 1-41. Illustration of anatomic injury zones for the extensor tendons.

At the level of the extensor retinaculum the extensor tendons are enclosed in tendon sheaths.[23,35] Just proximal to the metacarpophalangeal joints, the extensor digitorum communis tendons are joined together by interconnections (juncturae tendinum) (Fig. 1-39).[23] At the level of the metacarpophalangeal joint, the extensor tendons are stabilized by the conjoined tendons of the intrinsic muscles of the hand and the sagittal band (Fig. 1-39).[23,35] The sagittal band arises from the volar plate and collateral ligaments.[23,35]

At the proximal interphalangeal joint, the extensor tendon is stabilized by three slips. The central slip attaches to the dorsal distal middle phalanx and two slips that span the joint to attach on the dorsal distal phalanx (Fig. 1-40).[23,35]

It is important that injury to the tendons and supporting structures is evaluated with high-resolution axial and sagittal MRI, especially in the hand.[11] Therefore, like the flexor tendons, zones have been developed for surgical treatment planning (Fig. 1-41).[19,20,42]

NEUROVASCULAR ANATOMY

The neurovascular anatomy of the hand and wrist is complex. The vascular anatomy is important for soft-tissue injury, fracture healing and avascular necrosis.[11] There are numerous causes of nerve compression, so it is essential to understand neurovascular and related anatomy in the hand and wrist.[3,21,22,45,46]

Vascular Anatomy

The vascular anatomy of the hand and wrist can be demonstrated on conventional sequences and image planes or with MR angiography.[11] The vascular supply to the hand and wrist (Fig. 1-42) can be divided into extrinsic and intrinsic.

The extrinsic supply is derived from branches of the radial, ulnar, and anterior interosseous arteries. The radial and ulnar arteries form the margins of three dorsal and palmar anastomotic arcades.[14,35] The most proximal arcades lie palmar and dorsal to the radiocarpal joint. The second arcade is palmar and dorsal to the intercarpal joints and the most distal are the dorsal basal and deep palmar arches.[14,35]

The intrinsic vascular supply is critical for bone healing and involves distal branches of the extrinsic vessels that supply the osseous structures of the wrist.[18,32] The carpal bones have been divided into three groups based on the vascular supply. Group I carpal bones have only one surface entry point and so are more susceptible to ischemic changes. This group includes the scaphoid, capitate, and 20% of lunate bones.[32] Group II carpal bones have at least two points of arterial entry but no intraosseous anastomoses. The trapezoid and hamate bones are included with this group. Group III carpal bones have multiple arterial entry points with intraosseous anastomoses. The trapezium, triquetrum, pisiform, and 80% of lunate bones fall into this category.[14,32]

Distal to the palmar arch, the common digital arteries extend to the level of the metacarpophalangeal joints where they branch to send proper digital arteries along the margins of each digit (Fig. 1-42).[11]

Neural Anatomy

On the ulnar side of the distal forearm proximal to the carpal tunnel, the ulnar artery, nerve, and the accompanying veins lie deep to the flexor carpi ulnaris (Fig. 1-43).[30,33,35] The nerve is generally medial to the artery at this level. At the level of the pisiform, these structures pass along the lateral or radial side of the pisiform, passing deep to the volar carpal ligament and then distally into the palm of the hand anterior to the flexor retinaculum but deep to the palmaris brevis muscle (Fig. 1-43).[11,25,30,33] At the level of the pisiform, the ulnar nerve typically divides into superficial and deep branches. In addition, at the pisiform level, the nerve and accompanying vascular structures lie between the volar carpal ligament and flexor retinaculum in a space commonly known as Guyon's canal (Fig. 1-44). Lesions proximal to or within the canal can produce both sensory and motor abnormalities in the ulnar nerve distribution.[30,33,34]

The two-flexor digitorum muscles (superficial and profundus) are lateral to the ulnar nerve and vessels at the level of the wrist. The tendon of the palmaris longus lies superficially (Fig. 1-43). These structures are most easily identified

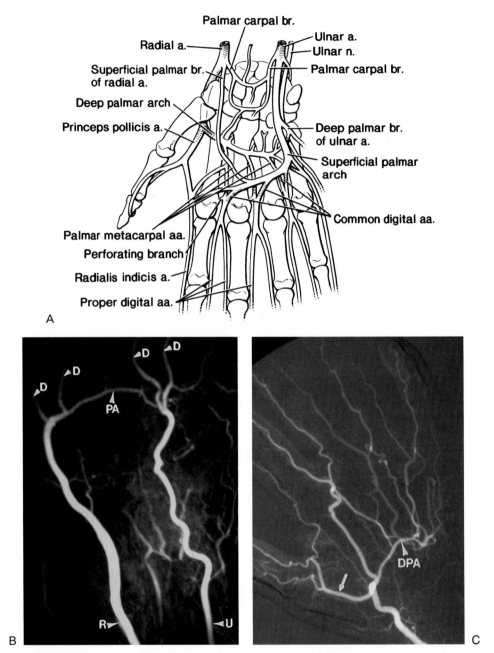

FIGURE 1-42. A: Illustration of the vascular anatomy of the hand and wrist. (From Berquist TH. MRI of the musculoskeletal system, 4th ed. Philadelphia: Lippincott Williams & Wilkins, 2001:733–841.) **B:** MR angiogram demonstrating the radial (R) and ulnar (U) arteries, superficial palmar arch (PA), and digital arteries (D). **C:** Selective radial artery injection demonstrating the deep palmar arch (DPA), princeps pollicis artery *(arrow),* and digital arteries to the hand.

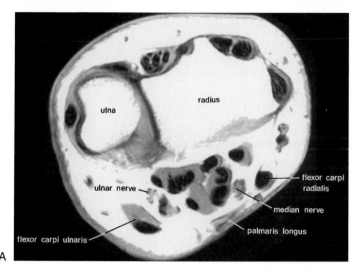

A

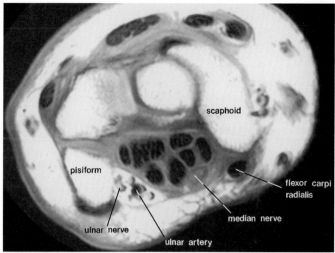

B

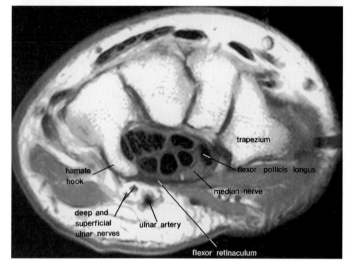

C

FIGURE 1-43. Axial MR images demonstrating the relationships of the ulnar and median nerves at the level of the distal radioulnar joint **(A)** and pisiform **(B),** and hamate hook **(C).**

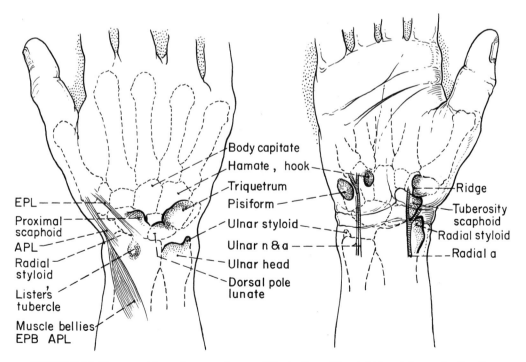

FIGURE 1-44. Topographic anatomy and coronal illustration of the right hand demonstrating the relationship of the ulnar nerve to the pisiform and hamate hook.

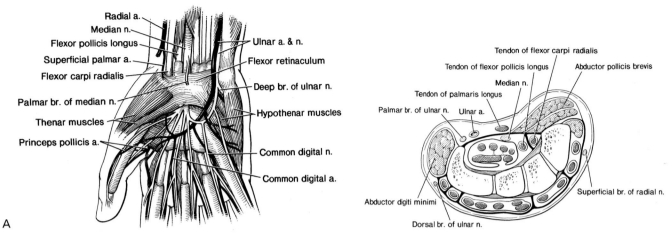

FIGURE 1-45. Illustrations of the neurovascular anatomy of the hand and wrist **(A)** and axial illustration of the carpal tunnel **(B)**. (From Berquist TH. MRI of the musculoskeletal system, 4th ed. Philadelphia: Lippincott Williams & Wilkins, 2001:773–841.)

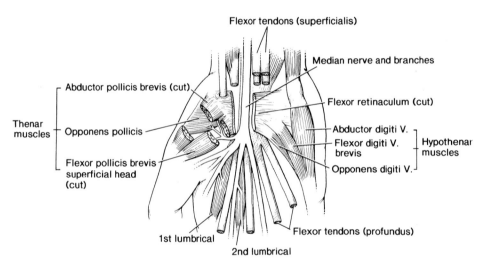

FIGURE 1-46. Illustration of the median nerve and its branches. (From Berquist TH. MRI of the musculoskeletal system, 4th ed. Philadelphia: Lippincott Williams & Wilkins, 2001:773–841.)

on axial MR images. The midline volar structures of the wrist, as they enter the carpal tunnel, tend to form three layers. The most superficial or anterior layer is formed by the flexor digitorum superficialis. The middle layer is formed by the superficial flexor of the index and middle fingers, and the most posterior or deepest layer is formed by the flexor digitorum profundus tendons. All tendons have a common sheath just before they pass under the flexor retinaculum. The palmaris longus tendon is the most superficial and midline structure at the wrist level (Figs. 1-43A and 1-45).

The median nerve lies deep to the flexor digitorum superficialis through much of the forearm. Just proximal to the wrist, it emerges on the radial side of the superficial flexor and passes forward and medially to lie in front of the flexor tendons in the carpal tunnel (Fig. 1-46).[26] At the distal margin of the flexor retinaculum, the median nerve divides into five or six branches. These small branches are difficult to identify, even when thin axial MR sections are obtained.[1,25]

REFERENCES

1. Anderson MW, Kaplan PA, Dussault RG, et al. Magnetic resonance imaging of the wrist. Curr Probl Diagn Radiol 1998; Nov/Dec:189–226.
2. Arons MS, Fishbone G, Arons JA. Communicating defects of the triangular fibrocartilage complex without disruption of the triangular fibrocartilage: a report of 2 cases. J Hand Surg 1999; 24A:148–151.
3. Baker LL, Hajek PC, Björkengren A, et al. High resolution magnetic resonance imaging of the wrist: normal anatomy. Skel Radiol 1987;16:128–132.
4. Berger RA. General anatomy. In: Cooney WP III, Linscheid RL, Dobyns JH, eds. The wrist: diagnosis and operative treatment. St. Louis: Mosby, 1998:32–60.
5. Berger RA. Ligament anatomy. In: Cooney WP III, Linscheid RL, Dobyns JH, eds. The wrist: diagnosis and operative treatment. St. Louis: Mosby, 1998:73–105.
6. Berger RA, Kauer JMG, Landsmeer JMF. Radioscapholunate ligament: A gross anatomic and histologic study of fetal and adult wrists. J Hand Surg 1991;16A:350–355.
7. Berger RA, Landsmeer JMF. The palmar radiocarpal ligaments: A study of adult and fetal human wrist joints. J Hand Surg 1990;15A:847–854.
8. Berger RA. The gross and histologic anatomy of the scapholunate interosseous ligament. J Hand Surg 1996;21A:170–178.
9. Berquist TH. Imaging of orthopedic trauma, 2nd ed. New York: Raven Press, 1992:749–870.
10. Berquist TH. Magnetic resonance imaging of the elbow and wrist. Top Magn Reson Imaging 1989;1:15–27.
11. Berquist TH. MRI of the musculoskeletal system, 4th ed. Philadelphia: Lippincott Williams & Wilkins, 2001:773–841.
12. Boles CA, Kannams, Cardwell AB. The forearm anatomy of the muscle compartments and nerves. AJR 2000;174:151–159.
13. Brown RR, Fliszar E, Cotton A, et al. Extrinsic and intrinsic ligaments of the wrist: normal and pathologic anatomy at MR arthrography with three-compartment enhancement. Radiographics 1998;18:667–674.
14. Cooney WP. Vascular and neurologic anatomy of the wrist. In: Cooney WP III, Linscheid RL, Dobyns JH, eds. The wrist: diagnosis and operative treatment. St. Louis: Mosby, 1998:106–123.
15. Erickson SJ, Neeland JB, Middleton WD, et al. MR imaging

16. Garcia-Elias M, Dobyns JH. Bones and joints. In: Cooney WP III, Linscheid RL, Dobyns JH. The wrist: diagnosis and operative treatment. St. Louis: Mosby, 1998:61–72.
17. Garcia-Elias M, An K-N, Cooney WP III, et al. Stability of the transverse arch: an experimental study. J Hand Surg 1989;14A:277–282.
18. Gelberman RH, Panagis JS, Taleisnik J, et al. The arterial anatomy of the human carpus. Part I: The extraosseous vascularity. J Hand Surg 1983;8A:367–375.
19. Ham SJ, Konings JG, Wolf RFE, et al. Functional anatomy of the soft tissues of the hand and wrist. In vivo excursion measurement of the flexor pollicis longus tendon using MRI. Magn Reson Imaging 1993;11:163–167.
20. Hauger O, Chung CB, Lektrakul N, et al. Pulley system in the fingers: normal anatomy and simulated lesions in cadavers at MR imaging, CT and US with and without contrast material distension of the tendon sheath. Radiology 2000;217:201–212.
21. Hayman LA, Duncan G, Chiou-Tan FY, et al. Sectional anatomy of the upper limb III: Forearm and hand. J Compt Asst Tomogr 2001;25(2):322–325.
22. Ikeda K, Haughton VM, Ho K-C, et al. Correlative MR anatomy of the median nerve. AJR 1996;167:1233–1236.
23. Kaplan PA. Anatomy, injuries, and treatment of the extensor apparatus of the hand and fingers. Clin Orthop 1959;13:24–41.
24. Keir PJ, Wells RP. Changes in geometry of the finger flexor tendons in the carpal tunnel with the wrist posture and tendon load: an MRI study of normal wrists. Clin Biomechanics 1999;14:635–645.
25. Mäuver J, Bleschkowski A, Tempka A, et al. High-resolution MR imaging of the carpal tunnel and the wrist. Acta Radiologica 2000;41:78–83.
26. Mesgarzadeh M, Schneck CD, Bonakdapour A. Carpal tunnel: MR imaging. Part I: Normal anatomy. Radiology 1989;171:743–748.
27. Middleton WD, Macronder S, Lawson TL, et al. High resolution surface coil magnetic resonance imaging of the joints. Anatomic correlation. Radiographics 1987;7:645–683.
28. Mikic ZD. Age related changes in the triangular fibrocartilage of the wrist joint. J Anat 1978;126:367–384.
29. Mikic ZD. Arthrography of the wrist joint. An experimental study. J Bone Joint Surg 1984;66A:371–378.
30. Netcher D, Polsen C, Thomby J, et al. Anatomic delineation of the ulnar nerve and artery in relation to the carpal tunnel by axial magnetic resonance imaging scanning. J Hand Surg 1996;21A:273–276.
31. Palmer AK, Werner FW. The triangular fibrocartilage complex of the wrist: anatomy and function. J Hand Surg 1981;61:153–162.
32. Panagis JS, Gelberman RH, Taleisnik J, et al. The arterial anatomy of the human carpus. II: The intraosseous vascularity. J Hand Surg 1983;8A:375–382.
33. Pierre-Jerome C, Bekkelund SI, Nordstrom R. Quantitative MRI analysis of anatomic dimensions of the carpal tunnel in women. J Clin Anat 1997;19:31–34.
34. Pretorius ES, Epstein RE, Dalinka MK. MR imaging of the wrist. Radiol Clin N Am 1997;35:145–161.
35. Rosse C, Rosse PC. Hollingsheads textbook of anatomy. Philadelphia: Lippincott–Raven Publishers, 1997:239–309.
36. Schimmel-Metz SM, Metz VM, Totterman SMS, et al. Radiologic measurement of the scapholunate joint: implications of biologic variation in scapholunate joint morphology. J Hand Surg 1999;24A:1237–1244.
37. Smith DK, Snearly WN. Lunotriquetral interosseous ligament of the wrist: MR appearances in asymptomatic volunteers

and arthrographically normal wrists. Radiology 1994;191:199–202.

38. Smith DK. Anatomic fractures of the carpal scaphoid: validation of biometric measurements and symmetry with three-dimensional MR imaging. Radiology 1993;187:187–191.

39. Smith DK. Scapholunate interosseous ligament of the wrist: MR appearances in asymptomatic volunteers and arthrographically normal wrists. Radiology 1994;192:217–221.

40. Smith DK. Volar carpal ligaments of the wrist. Normal appearance on multiplanar reconstruction of three-dimensional Fourier transform MR images. AJR 1993;161:353–357.

41. Theumann NH, Pfirrmann CWA, Trudell DJ, et al. MR imaging of the metacarpophalangeal joint of the fingers. Conventional MR imaging and MR arthrographic findings in cadavers. Radiology 2002;222:431–445.

42. Totterman SMS, Miller RJ. Triangular fibrocartilage complex: normal appearance on coronal three-dimensional gradient recalled echo MR images. Radiology 1995;195:521–527.

43. Verdan C. Tendon surgery of the hand. Edinburgh: Churchill Livingstone, 1979:57–66.

44. Viegas SF, Wagner K, Patterson R, et al. Medial hamate facet of the lunate. J Hand Surg 1990;15A:564–571.

45. Viegas SF, Crossley M, Marzke M, et al. The fourth carpometacarpal joint. J Hand Surg 1991;16A:525–533.

46. Weiss KL, Beltran J, Shamon OM, et al. High-field MR surface-coil imaging in the hand and wrist. I: Normal anatomy. Radiology 1986;260:143–146.

47. Zeiss J, Skie M, Ebraheim N, et al. Anatomic relations between the median nerve and flexor tendons in the carpal tunnel: MR evaluations in normal volunteers. AJR 1989;153:533–536.

2

MAGNETIC RESONANCE IMAGING TECHNIQUES

THOMAS H. BERQUIST
KIMBERLY K. AMRAMI

Imaging of the hand and wrist can be difficult due to the complex skeletal and soft-tissue anatomy. Optimization of numerous imaging techniques and approaches is important in today's cost-conscious environment.[1,6] Routine radiographs or computed radiography images are usually adequate for detection of fractures and osseous pathology. Fluoroscopically positioned spot views are useful in subtle cases to assure optimal positioning and reduce bony overlap.[6,27] Subtle changes may require radionuclide studies or computed tomography (CT) to clearly define the nature of osseous lesions. Ultrasonography is useful for evaluating the soft tissues and joints, as well as for differentiating solid from cystic soft-tissue masses. Invasive studies, such as arthrography, tonography, and angiography, may also be useful.[6,7]

The role of magnetic resonance imaging (MRI) has continued to expand as pulse sequencing and high-resolution imaging, including new 3.0 Tesla (3T) imaging, arthrographic, and angiographic techniques, have improved.[3,6,18,25,39]

Recent studies have demonstrated that MRI has significant usefulness and impacts clinical decisions regarding a significant number of patients.[22,23] Hobby et al.[23] demonstrated that MR studies changed the clinical diagnosis in 55%, changed the treatment plan in 45%, and improved the physicians' understanding of the disease process in 67% of patients.

PATIENT SELECTION

Several basic factors must be considered when selecting patients for MRI. These include patient safety factors, patient size, suspected pathology, need for premedication (for pain, claustrophobia, or children), and efficacy.[6,13]

The Safety Committee of the International Society of Magnetic Resonance in Medicine recommended standard policies for patient safety and screening.[9,13] A written questionnaire along with verbal questions should be completed prior to the examination.[6,9] This should prevent the oversight of obvious risk factors, such as cardiac pacemakers, cerebral aneurysm clips, metallic foreign bodies, or electrical devices that may place the patient at risk during the examination.[6,9] When metallic foreign bodies are suspected, the area should be studied with radiography or CT prior to the MR examination.[6,9,13]

Magnetic fields may affect certain metal implants and electrical devices. Each MR suite should have references for these materials.[6,34] Metallic fixation devices and prostheses are configured of high-grade stainless steel or alloys that may cause artifacts and local image distortion. The degree of image degradation depends on the type of metal, configuration, and size of the device. Though most internal devices used in the hand and wrist are small, the local image distortion may still be too great to evaluate the complex anatomy (Fig. 2-1). Cast materials restrict positioning and may require use of a larger coil but do not reduce image quality.[6]

The patient's age, clinical status, and type and length of examination must be considered to determine if sedation, anesthesia, or pain medication will be required. Patients can be safely monitored during MR examination.[6]

Anxious patients or patients with significant pain or inability to maintain necessary positions may not be able to tolerate potentially lengthy MR examinations. Children younger than 6 years may not be able to cooperate sufficiently to obtain an optimal examination. A parent or friend may accompany the patient into the examination suite to reduce anxiety or to assist a child during the study. In certain cases, sedation or medication may be required.[6] Patients requiring pain medication or sedation should be screened for risk factors (asthma, chronic lung disease, cardiovascular disease, and so forth).

Sedation may be divided into several categories depending on the patient's status and type of sedation required. Conscious sedation is a pharmacologically induced state of depressed consciousness that permits the patient to respond to verbal commands. Deep sedation is similar to general anesthesia, and patients are not easily aroused.[16] The medication selected is based on clinical status and the level of sedation required.[16,20]

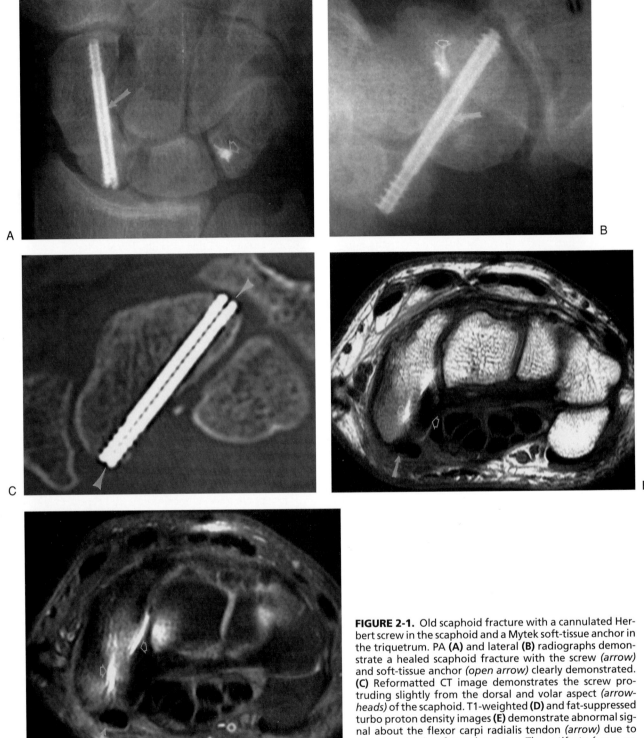

FIGURE 2-1. Old scaphoid fracture with a cannulated Herbert screw in the scaphoid and a Mytek soft-tissue anchor in the triquetrum. PA **(A)** and lateral **(B)** radiographs demonstrate a healed scaphoid fracture with the screw *(arrow)* and soft-tissue anchor *(open arrow)* clearly demonstrated. **(C)** Reformatted CT image demonstrates the screw protruding slightly from the dorsal and volar aspect *(arrowheads)* of the scaphoid. T1-weighted **(D)** and fat-suppressed turbo proton density images **(E)** demonstrate abnormal signal about the flexor carpi radialis tendon *(arrow)* due to chronic irritation from the screw. The artifacts *(open arrows)* are minimal in this case.

When possible, oral sedation is preferred. Chloral hydrate is an effective oral sedation for children, especially for those under 2 years of age.[8,20] Chloral hydrate can be administered incrementally. In patients older than 1 year, oral hydroxyzine can be added. In patients aged 2 to 4 years, some pediatricians recommend meperidine intramuscularly when the above approaches fail.[16,37] Greenberg et al.[20] reported excellent results when combining chloral hydrate (50 to 100 mg/kg 30 minutes before examination) with thioridazine (2 to 4 mg/kg 2 hours before examination) in pediatric patients who were difficult to sedate.

Intravenous sedation or pain medications require patient monitoring, but the onset and effects are more predictable. We use midazolam, fentanyl, and, for the elderly, diphenhydramine for intravenous sedation. The type of intravenous sedation used varies with the patient's status, length of examination, and physician preference.[6,9,16]

Patients who have been sedated, specifically deeply sedated, must be observed after the procedure. Before discharge, patients should be stable, be easily aroused, have reflexes intact, and be able to communicate accurately.[16] Children can be dismissed to a parent or guardian. Adults should not be allowed to drive for 24 hours. Therefore, another adult must accompany them if they must travel after the procedure.

PATIENT POSITIONING/COIL SELECTION

Magnetic resonance examinations of the hand and wrist require exceptional anatomic detail. This can be difficult to accomplish due to limitations in positioning and reduced patient comfort. Patient comfort is essential to prevent motion artifact and image degradation.[1,6]

Positioning depends on patient size, information required (motion studies, etc.), software, and coil availability. When possible, we position the patient supine with the wrist at the side. This is generally the most comfortable position for the patient (Fig. 2-2). The wrist can also be placed over the abdomen with the elbow flexed. However, the coil must be supported and separated from the abdominal wall to prevent respiratory motion artifact. Larger patients and children may be positioned prone or in the lateral decubitus position with the arm above the head (Fig. 2-3). In this setting, shoulder discomfort and motion artifact are common problems.[1,6]

Once the wrist is positioned, it should be supported with foam pads or bolsters to reduce motion and enhance comfort. The exception to this approach is when motion studies are required. In this case, motion control devices can be used to optimize position changes.[1,2,6,24,36]

Coils for hand and wrist imaging (Fig. 2-4) are available in multiple configurations (flat, circular, wrap-around, partial volume, and circumferential).[6,18,26,28,38,40] Coil selection

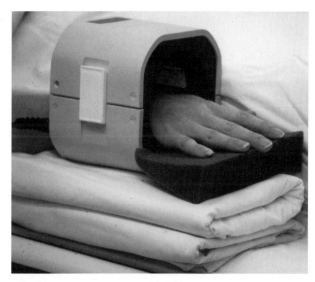

FIGURE 2-2. Patient positioning. Photograph of a patient with the arm at the side, the hand prone in a wrist coil supported with towels.

varies with the clinical indications and position or positions required. Circular 3-in. or 5-in. coils are useful when motion studies are performed, as there is more latitude for position changes. Dual coils can be used to study both hands and wrists when pathology is bilateral or when comparison is required.[21]

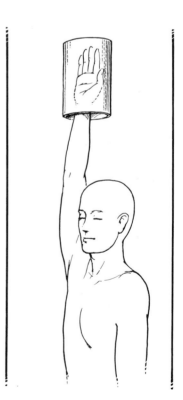

FIGURE 2-3. Illustration of a patient positioned with the arm above the head. The wrist is in the center of the bore using a circumferential coil.

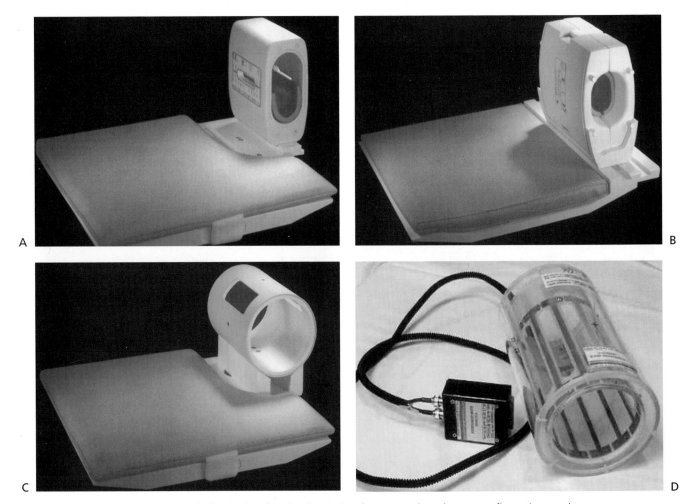

FIGURE 2-4. Coils for the hand and wrist. **A:** Quadrature or phased array configuration can be positioned at the patient's side or overhead, either vertically or horizontally. Hand and wrist coil. **B:** Four-channel phased array for the wrist can be used with ≤6 cm field of view. Coil can be used at the patient's side, overhead and in vertical or horizontal positions. **C:** Small extremity quadrature or phased-array coil. (A–C can be used with GE or Siemens systems. Courtesy of MRI Devices Corp., Waukesha, Wisconsin.) **D:** BC-10 (Birdcage 10 cm) coil for hand and wrist imaging at 3T. (Coil design by Joel Felmlee, PhD, with postdoctoral study Armen Kocharian, PhD, Mayo Clinic, Rochester, Minnesota.)

To achieve high spatial resolution, a small field of view (FOV) of 8 to 12 cm is routinely employed. The image matrix should be 256 to 512 with 1- to 3-mm-thick sections. Smaller sections (0.6 to 1 mm) are used for volume acquisitions and three-dimensional studies.[6,35] In general, one acquisition is adequate.[6]

Most imaging of the hand and wrist is performed at 1.5 Tesla (T). However, experience with 3.0-T magnets is increasing. The primary advantage of extremity imaging at 3.0 T lies in the increased signal-to-noise ratio (SNR) at 3.0 T compared with lower field strengths. SNR increases linearly with field strength; hence, the SNR at 3.0 T is twice that of standard systems at 1.5 T. This allows significant improvements in spatial resolution without increasing imaging time, providing more detailed anatomic imaging of the small, often

out-of-plane structures critical to advanced hand and wrist imaging. These include the extrinsic and intrinsic ligaments of the wrist, the triangular fibrocartilage complex, articular cartilage, neurovascular structures, and the fine ligamentous structures of the hands (Fig. 2-5).

We have used custom-made transmit/receive coils (birdcage type) (Fig. 2-4D) successfully for extremity imaging at 3.0 T, typically with a 6-cm internal diameter for fingers and a 10-cm internal diameter for hand and wrist. This has resulted in even greater improvements in SNR when compared with traditional phased-array coils. The use of birdcage coils also does not require the use of the body coil as a transmitter, substantially reducing the amount of radiofrequency (RF) power needed and limiting the RF effects to the extremity under study. MRI at higher field strengths (3.0 to

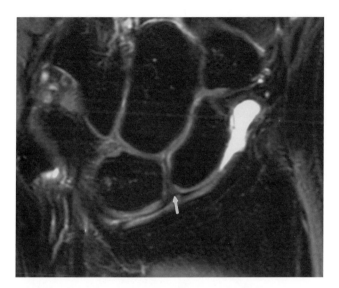

FIGURE 2-5. 3T coronal fast spin echo with fat saturation (3500/80, ET12, 2-mm section, 10 cm field of view, 256 × 256, 3 Nex) clearly demonstrates the articular cartilage and scapholunate ligament *(arrow)*. Fluid is high signal intensity.

4.0 T) may offer major advantages over imaging at 1.5 T and below in the musculoskeletal system, particularly in complex areas such as the wrist and fingers.

PULSE SEQUENCES/IMAGE PLANES

There are numerous pulse sequences and image planes that can be selected for imaging studies of the hand and wrist.[6,14,15,30] High resolution and optimal image quality are essential.

The sequences and image planes selected vary with clinical indication. We perform a standard screening examination in most cases (Table 2-1) and add additional sequences or gadolinium when indicated. T1-weighted sequences are useful for osseous anatomy, marrow, delineation of fat planes

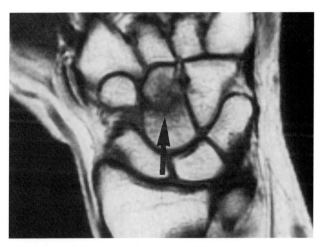

FIGURE 2-6. Coronal T1-weighted (SE 500/10) image of the wrist demonstrates low signal intensity in the capitate *(arrow)* due to a fracture and surrounding marrow edema.

and fatty masses, and for hemorrhage (increased signal on T1-weighted image) (Fig. 2-6).[1,6] Pathologic processes and joint fluid have high signal intensity on T2-weighted sequences (Fig. 2-7A). These sequences provide excellent contrast between pathology and muscle or cortical bone. Fat signal intensity is suppressed with this pulse sequence. The same is true for fast spin echo (FSE) T2-weighted sequences. The FSE sequences can be performed more quickly, and there is less image degradation by motion artifact. We use fat suppression technique with FSE sequences to avoid overlooking marrow and soft-tissue abnormalities, as both have high intensity similar to fluid. Fat suppression results in a low intensity for marrow and fat, so that presence of fluid, edema, and other pathologic changes are easily detected (Fig. 2-7B).[6,10,18]

Conventional short T1 inversion recovery (STIR) sequences have been replaced by FSE inversion recovery techniques (Table 2-1). Fluid and pathologic conditions have high signal intensity in comparison with suppressed marrow and soft tissues.[1,6]

TABLE 2-1. HAND AND WRIST IMAGING PROTOCOLS[6,25,38]

Procedure	Plane	Sequence	TE/TR	FOV (cm)	Matrix	Slice/Gap (mm)	Nex
Screening examination	Coronal	T1	450/10	8	256 × 256	3/0.3	2
	Coronal	T2	2000/20,80	8	256 × 256	3/0.3	1
	Coronal	3D-GRE	45/9,30°	8	256 × 256	1/60/100	1
	Axial	FSE IR	3000/80/150	8	256 × 256	3/1	1
	Axial	T1	450/10	8	256 × 256	3/1	2
	Sagittal	FSE PD FS	4000/20, ET8	8	256 × 224	3/1	2
Wrist arthrography *(0.2 cm³*	Coronal	T1 FS	650/18	8	256 × 256	3/0.5	2
Gad in 20 cm³ of iodinated	Sagittal	T1 FS	650/18	8	256 × 256	3/0.5	2
contrast ± lidocaine and	Axial	T1 FS	650/18	8	256 × 256	3/0.5	2
celestone)	Coronal	3D-GRE	45/9, 30°	8	256 × 192	1/60/0.5	1
Hand and wrist MR angiography *(0.2 mm/kg IV)*	Coronal	3D-GRE	21/6, 30° or 3.8/1.4, 30° if available	25	256 × 512	1/40	1

FOV, field of view; FSE, fast spin echo; FS, fat suppression; GRE, gradient recalled echo.

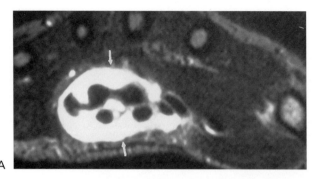

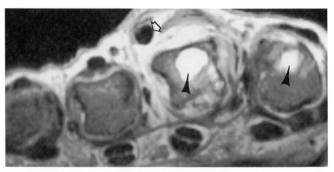

A

B

FIGURE 2-7. T2-weighted sequences. **A:** Axial image (SE 2000/80) demonstrating high signal intensity fluid *(arrows)* about the flexor tendons due to tenosynovitis. **B:** Fast spin echo T2-weighted axial image with fat suppression demonstrates low signal intensity marrow in the metacarpal heads with high signal intensity in the geodes *(arrowheads)* and inflamed soft tissues. Note the subluxed extensor tendon *(open arrow)*.

Gradient echo sequences (Fig. 2-8) can be performed using conventional two-dimensional or three-dimensional volume acquisitions. We use the latter with sixty 0.6- to 1-mm sections (Table 2-1) to allow reformatting in any image plane. Ligament, capsular, and articular anatomy are well defined with this approach.[6,35]

We are currently evaluating a dual-echo steady state (DESS) sequence for evaluating articular cartilage. This sequence is a volume water excitation sequence that results in low signal intensity for marrow (fat suppression) and high signal intensity for articular cartilage (Fig. 2-9). Multiple (about 100) 1-mm sections can be obtained using this sequence. Scan time is 6 minutes and 26 seconds.

Our screening examination includes images in all three planes and multiplanar reformatting with the gradient echo sequence (Table 2-1). Table 2-2 summarizes image planes by anatomic region (Fig. 2-10).[1,6,18]

Gadolinium is a paramagnetic ion with seven unpaired electrons that has gained popularity due to efficiency in

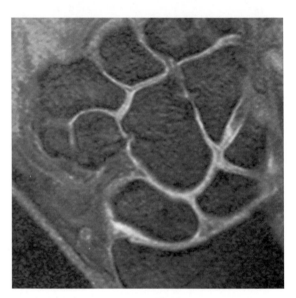

FIGURE 2-9. Coronal dual-echo steady state (DESS) sequence demonstrates low marrow signal with high intensity articular cartilage (23.87/6.73, FA 25°, ET1, 256 × 256, 1 acquisition, 12 cm field of view, 1-mm-thick sections).

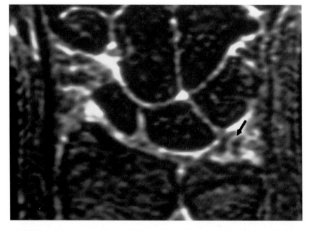

FIGURE 2-8. Coronal gradient echo (45/9, 30°) image demonstrating a tear *(arrow)* in the triangular fibrocartilage.

TABLE 2-2. MRI OF THE HAND AND WRIST: IMAGE PLANES

Anatomic Structure	Image Plane
Distal radius and ulna	Axial and coronal
	Sagittal for fragment alignment
Distal radioulnar joint	Coronal
	Axial (neutral, pronation, supination)
Soft-tissue proximal wrist	Axial and sagittal
Carpal tunnel	Axial
Carpal bones—scaphoid	Axial and coronal
	Add oblique sagittal
Metacarpals/phalanges	Axial, oblique sagittal
Tendons	Axial and sagittal
Ligaments	Axial, coronal, oblique reformats

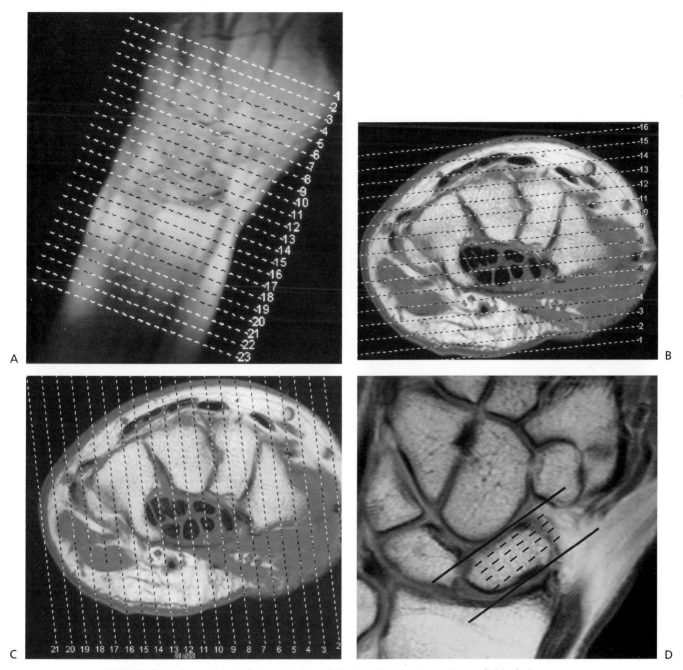

FIGURE 2-10. Image plane for evaluation of the hand and wrist. **A:** Large field of view coronal T1-scout image for selection of conventional axial images of the wrist and proximal hand. **B:** T1-weighted axial scout for selection of conventional coronal images. **C:** T1-weighted axial scout for selection of conventional sagittal images. **D, E:** Coronal T1-weighted image **(D)** with oblique sagittal sections selected. Fat-suppressed enhanced sagittal image **(E)** demonstrating the scaphoid (S). (*Figure continues.*)

T1 shortening and the relative lack of side effects. To avoid toxic side effects, gadolinium has been chelated to several substances, including dimeglumine (gadolinium dimeglumine), tetraazacyclododecanetetraacetic acid, and diethylenetriaminepentaacetic acid. In most cases, 0.1 mL/kg is injected. Nephrotoxicity is less than with iodinated contrast agents.[5,6,31]

Gadolinium is not routinely used for hand and wrist imaging. However, the applications continue to expand using intravenous gadolinium for enhancing pathology and angiographic techniques.[6,25,39] Intra-articular gadolinium (MR arthrography) is also performed commonly at our institution. MR tenography has not become commonplace in our practice.

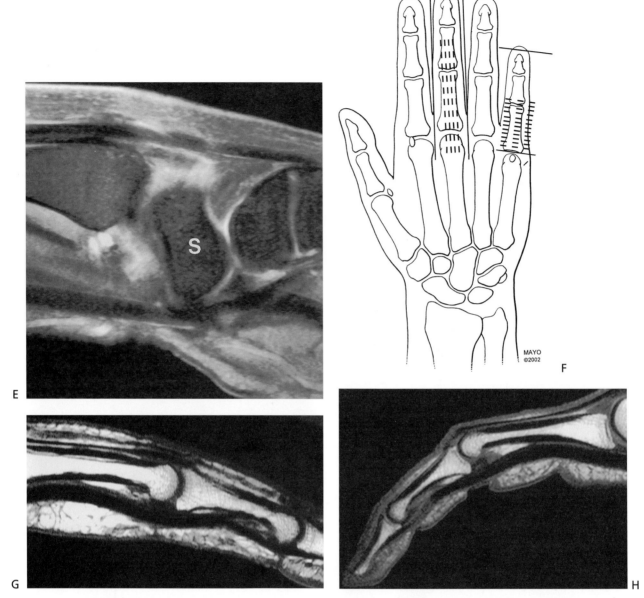

FIGURE 2-10. (*continued*) **F–H:** Illustration of the hand and wrist demonstrating **(F)** axial image plane selection for the fifth finger and sagittal images of the third finger. Sagittal T1-weighted images through the flexor tendon in extension **(G)** and slight flexion **(H)**.

INTRAVENOUS GADOLINIUM

Gadolinium remains intravascular for a short period before being distributed to intracellular fluid. Areas of inflammation, neoplasms, and other pathologic tissues enhance rapidly and retain contrast longer than normal tissues.[5,29] Contrast studies are also useful for evaluating flow in patients with fractures, suspected avascular necrosis, or nonunion.[6,11] Techniques for intravenous injection vary with suspected pathology. In most cases, precontrast T1- and T2-weighted images are obtained. Postcontrast fat-suppressed T1-weighted images are obtained after injection.

Gradient echo sequences can be used for dynamic studies for suspected neoplasms.[5,6] Image planes are usually performed in the same two planes after contrast to permit image comparison.[6]

Intravenous gadolinium can also be useful for the management of articular disorders (Fig. 2-11). Enhancement of synovium occurs with arthropathies as early as 10 minutes after injection. Enhancement of synovium and joint fluid increases over time, so that images can be obtained for up to 1 hour after injection.[5,6] Inflamed ligaments and tendons also enhance, which may be confused with disruption of these structures.[6]

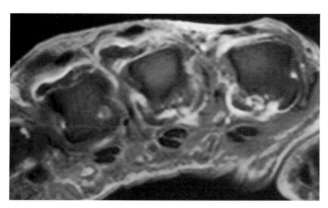

FIGURE 2-11. Axial fat-suppressed T-1 weighted, contrast-enhanced image demonstrates inflamed synovium in the metacarpophalangeal joints.

MR ARTHROGRAPHY

Wrist and hand arthrograms can be performed using indirect (intravenous) or intra-articular approaches.

Indirect arthrography has several advantages in that it is minimally invasive, enhances the joint fluid effect, does not require additional time for fluoroscopic injection, and permits the use of faster, fat-suppressed, T1-weighted sequences (Fig. 2-11).[33] Though fluid in all compartments enhances, Schweitzer et al.[33] reported accuracy of 100% for triangular fibrocartilage tears and 96% for scapholunate ligament tears. Passive or active exercise is performed prior to imaging the wrist to enhance uniform fluid distribution.[6,33]

Disadvantages of indirect arthrography include lack of fluid control (cannot measure capsule size), inability to aspirate fluid for laboratory studies, inability to inject anesthetic and/or steroid for diagnostic therapeutic purposes, and in-ability to do isolated compartment studies (Fig. 2-11).[6,33] The last may make subtle lesions more difficult to detect.[6]

Intra-articular injections can be performed by palpation or with ultrasound or fluoroscopic guidance.[4,6,19] We prefer to do fluoroscopically guided studies with iodinated contrast and gadolinium, as changes may be evident during injection or with initial films prior to MRI.[6] The radiocarpal, intercarpal, and distal radioulnar joints may all need to be injected.[32,36] We start with the most symptomatic region or area of suspected pathology.[6]

The patient may be seated next to the fluoroscopic table or may lie supine with the arm extended and the hand palm down. The wrist is prepared using sterile technique and the entry site injected with local anesthetic (1% lidocaine) using a 25-gauge needle. The radiocarpal joint is entered dorsally with the wrist slightly flexed (Fig. 2-12). The entry site should be chosen to avoid the extensor tendons or scapholunate ligament region. The needle should be angled proximally to avoid the radial lip (Fig. 2-12). Three to four milliliters of contrast (0.2 cm^3 of gadolinium in 20 cm^3 of iodinated contrast with lidocaine) is injected under fluoroscopic observation. Injection of the intercarpal and distal radioulnar joints is performed with the hand flat using a direct vertical entry (Fig. 2-13).[6] Following the injection, the patient is moved to the MRI suite. The patient is positioned as described above. For conventional arthrography, a standard wrist or hand coil is used. When motion studies may be necessary, a positioning device to accurately change the degree of deviation or flexion and extension (5°/position change) and a noncircumferential coil is used.[17,24,36] For conventional MR arthrograms, we use pulse sequences as summarized in Table 2-1. Gradient echo sequences are used with motion studies with 3- to 4-mm sections through the wrist in each position.[6,36]

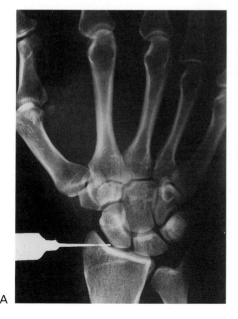

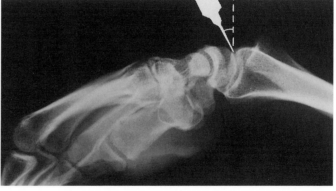

FIGURE 2-12. Illustration of injection site for the radiocarpal joint seen from dorsal **(A)** and lateral **(B)** views. Flexing the wrist slightly **(B)** facilitates the injection. The needle is angled proximally. The region of the scapholunate ligament should be avoided.

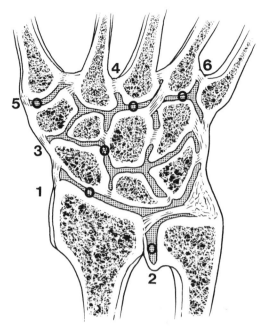

FIGURE 2-13. Illustration of the injection sites for the radiocarpal (1), distal radioulnar (2), and intercarpal joints (3). The common carpometacarpal (4), first carpometacarpal (5), and outer carpometacarpal (6) joints are rarely injected.

MR ANGIOGRAPHY

Magnetic resonance angiography of the hand and wrist may be performed with or without intravenous gadolinium.[6,25,39] Phase contrast (PC) and time of flight (TOF) techniques are performed without intravenous gadolinium. More recently, three-dimensional contrast-enhanced MR angiography has gained popularity.[25,39]

Time-of-Flight Technique

Flowing blood has high signal intensity using TOF techniques. Stationary protons become saturated following a series of RF pulses, whereas protons entering the region of RF stimulation are not saturated, resulting in greater longitudinal magnetization and increased signal intensity compared to the saturated protons.[6,25] Presaturation pulses can be used on either side of the section of interest to eliminate signal from flow, thereby selecting to evaluate either venous or arterial anatomy.[25,39]

The TOF sequences include both two- and three-dimensional approaches. Using the conventional two-dimensional approach, a series of overlapping thin sections are imaged to cover the area of interest. Three-dimensional studies may use volume (entire anatomic region stimulated) or multisection approaches.[25] The signal intensity and

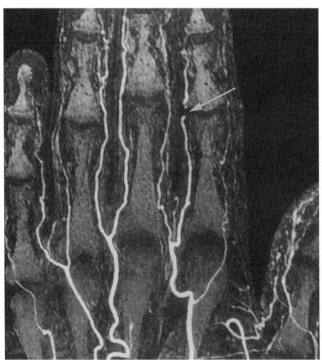

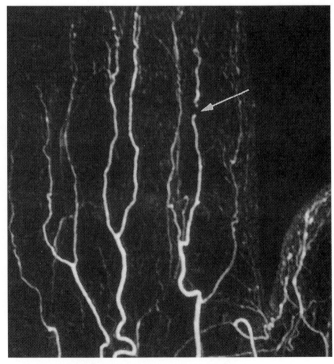

A   B

FIGURE 2-14. Contrast-enhanced MR angiogram. **A:** Unsubtracted image shows nonfilling of the ulnar digital artery at the proximal interphalangeal joint of the second digit *(arrow)* due to laceration and soft-tissue injury. **B:** Subtracted image shows the laceration defect *(arrow)* with refilling distally due to collaterals. (From Connell DA, Koulouris G, Thorn DA, et al. Contrast enhanced MR angiography of the hand. Radiographics 2002;22:583–599.)

contrast of flowing blood with all three techniques varies with repetition time and flip angle.

Phase Contrast Technique

Application of a second gradient pulse of equal magnitude and length can reverse the initial gradient pulse, which cancels the signal of stationary protons. Flowing blood is not affected in the same manner as stationary tissue, which results in a residual phase shift that is proportional to velocity.[6,25]

Phase contrast sequences have velocity-encoding factors that indicate the maximal flow velocity for which a given sequence is appropriate.

Both TOF and PC studies are turbulent flow and flow not perpendicular to the section being examined.[6,25,39]

Gadolinium-Enhanced MR Angiography

Contrast-enhanced, three-dimensional angiographic techniques have become increasingly popular in recent years.[12,39] Rapid acquisition data sets avoid the flow-sensitive issues seen with PC and TOF techniques.[39] Short acquisition times (<3 minutes) improve image quality and reduce venous filling, thereby allowing easier interpretation.[25] In fact, new three-dimensional sequences can be performed in less than 1 minute.[25,39] Unlike conventional hand and wrist imaging, a larger FOV (about 25 cm) is used so that the wrist and fingers can be included in the area studied.[25] Also, when necessary, both extremities can be studied simultaneously.[6] Use of precontrast three-dimensional sequences allows one to subtract the postcontrast images, resulting in greater vessel detail (Fig. 2-14).[12,25] Sequences used and contrast dose are summarized in Table 2-1.

Additional techniques may be required for specific clinical indications. These approaches will be discussed in subsequent chapters when they differ significantly from protocols described above (Table 2-1).

REFERENCES

1. Anderson MW, Kaplan PA, Dussault RG, et al. Magnetic resonance imaging of the wrist. Curr Probl Diagn Radiol 1998;Nov/Dec:187–219.
2. Azouz EM, Babyer PS, Mascia AT, et al. MRI of the abnormal pediatric hand and wrist with plain film correlation. J Comput Assist Tomogr 1998;22:252–261.
3. Baker LL, Hajek PC, Bjorkengren A, et al. High resolution magnetic resonance imaging of the wrist: normal anatomy. Skel Radiol 1987;16:128–132.
4. Beaulieu CF, Ladd AL. MR arthrography of the wrist: scanning room injection of the radiocarpal joint based on clinical landmarks. AJR 1998;170:606–608.
5. Beltran J, Chandnani V, McGhee RA, et al. Gadopentetate dimeglumine–enhanced MR imaging of the musculoskeletal system. AJR 1991;156:457–466.
6. Berquist TH. MRI of the musculoskeletal system, 4th ed. Philadelphia: Lippincott Williams & Wilkins, 2001:773–841.
7. Blain O, Binda R, Middleton W, et al. The occult dorsal carpal ganglion: usefulness of magnetic resonance imaging and ultrasound in diagnosis. Am J Orthop 1998;27(2):107–110.
8. Bloomfield EL, Masaryk TJ, Caplin A, et al. Intravenous sedation for MR imaging of the brain and spine in children: pentobarbital versus propofol. Radiology 1993;186:93–97.
9. Boutin RD, Briggs JE, Williamson MR. Injuries associated with MR imaging: safety records and methods used to screen patients for metallic foreign bodies before imaging. AJR 1994;162:189–194.
10. Brown RR, Fliszar E, Colten A, et al. Extrinsic and intrinsic ligaments of the wrist: normal and pathologic anatomy at MR arthrography with three-compartment enhancement. Radiographics 1998;18:687–774.
11. Cerezal L, Abuscal F, Canga A, et al. Usefulness of gadolinium-enhanced MR imaging in evaluation of the vascularity of scaphoid non-unions. AJR 2000;174:141–149.
12. Connell DA, Koulouris G, Thorn DA, et al. Contrast-enhanced MR angiography of the hand. Radiographics 2002;22:583–599.
13. Elster AD, Link KM, Carr JJ. Patient screening before MR imaging: a practical approach synthesized from protocols at 15 U.S. medical centers. AJR 1994;162:195–199.
14. Erickson SJ, Cox IH, Hyde JS, et al. Effect of tendon orientation on MR signal intensity: a manifestation of "magic angle" phenomenon. Radiology 1991;181:389–392.
15. Erickson SJ, Neeland JB, Middleton WD, et al. MR imaging of the finger: correlation with anatomic sections. AJR 1984;152:1013–1019.
16. Frush DP, Bissett GS III, Hall SC. Pediatric sedation in radiology: the practice of safe sleep. AJR 1996;167:1381–1387.
17. Gabl M, Lener M, Pechlaner S, et al. The role of dynamic magnetic resonance imaging in the detection of lesions of the ulnacarpal complex. J Hand Surg 1996;21B:311–314.
18. Girgis WS, Epstein RE. Magnetic resonance imaging of the hand and wrist. Semin Roentgenol 2000;35:286–296.
19. Grainger AJ, Elliott JM, Campbell RSD, et al. Direct MR arthrography: a review of current use. Clin Radiol 2000;55:163–176.
20. Greenberg SB, Falber EN, Radke JL, et al. Sedation of difficult to sedate children undergoing MR imaging. Value of thioridazine as an adjunct to chloral hydrate. AJR 1994;163:165–168.
21. Hardy CJ, Katzberg RW, Frey RL, et al. Switched surface coil system for bilateral MR imaging. Radiology 1988;167:835–838.
22. Hobby JL, Tom BDM, Bearcroft PWP, et al. Magnetic resonance imaging of the wrist: diagnostic performance statistics. Clin Radiol 2000;56:50–57.
23. Hobby JL, Dixon AK, Bearcroft PWP, et al. MR imaging of the wrist: effect on clinical diagnoses and patient care. Radiology 2001;220:589–593.
24. Kovanlikaya I, Camli D, Cakmakci H, et al. Diagnostic value of MR arthrography in detection of intrinsic carpal ligament lesions: use of cine-MR arthrography as a new approach. Eur Radiol 1997;7:1441–1445.
25. Lee VS, Lee HM, Rofsky NM. Magnetic resonance angiography of the hand. Invest. Radiol 1998;33(9):687–698.
26. Mauer J, Bleschkowski A, Templea A, et al. High-resolution MR imaging of the carpal tunnel and the wrist. Acta Radiol 2000;41:78–83.
27. Metz VM, Wunderbaldinger P, Gilula LA. Update on imaging techniques of the hand and wrist. Clin Plastic Surg 1996;23:369–384.
28. Middleton WD, Macrander S, Lawson TL, et al. High resolution surface coil magnetic resonance imaging of the joints: anatomic correlation. Radiographics 1987;7:645–683.

29. Nakahara R, Vetani M, Hayaski K, et al. Gadolinium enhanced MR imaging of the wrist in rheumatoid arthritis: value of fat suppressed pulse sequences. Skel Radiol 1996;25:639–647.

30. Parallada JA, Balkissoon ARA, Hayes CW, et al. Bowstring injury of the flexor tendon pulley system: MR imaging. AJR 1996;167:347–349.

31. Prince MR, Arnoldus C, Frisole JK. Nephrotoxicity of high dose gadolinium compared with iodinated contrast. J Magn Reson Imaging 1996;6:162–166.

32. Scheck RJ, Kubitzek C, Hierner R. The scapholunate interosseous ligament in MR arthrography of the wrist: correlation with non-enhanced MRI and wrist arthroscopy. Skel Radiol 1997;26:263–271.

33. Schweitzer ME, Natole P, Winalski CS, et al. Indirect wrist MR arthrography: the effect of passive motion versus active exercise. Skel Radiol 2000;29:10–14.

34. Shellock, FG. Pocket guide to MR procedures and metallic objects: update 1998. Philadelphia: Lippincott–Raven Publishers, 1998.

35. Smith DK. Dorsal carpal ligaments of the wrist: normal appearance on multiplanar reconstructions of three-dimensional Fourier transformed MR images. AJR 1993;161:119–125.

36. Tajiri Y, Nakamura K, Matshushita T, et al. A positioning device to allow rotation for cine-MRI of the distal radioulnar joint. Clin Radiol 1999;54:402–405.

37. Vade A, Sukhani R, Dolenga M, et al. Chloral hydrate sedation of children undergoing CT and MR imaging: safety as judged by the American Academy of Pediatrics Guidelines. AJR 1995;105:905–909.

38. Weiss KL, Beltran J, Shamam OM, et al. High-field surface coil imaging of the hand and wrist. I: Normal anatomy. Radiology 1986;160:143–146.

39. Winterer JT, Scheffler K, Paul G, et al. Optimization of contrast-enhanced MR angiography of the hands with a timing bolus and elliptically reordered 3D pulse sequence. J Comput Assist Tomogr 2000;24:903–908.

40. Wong EC, Jesmanowicz A, Hyde JS. High resolution short echo time MR imaging of the fingers and wrist with a local gradient coil. Radiology 1991;181:393–397.

PITFALLS

THOMAS H. BERQUIST

Pitfalls of magnetic resonance imaging (MRI) in the hand and wrist may be due to anatomic variants, improper technique, and software or hardware artifacts.[1,5]

Problems with patient motion, flow artifact, and other technical errors may result in suboptimal images. We have noted fewer problems with nonuniform fat suppression on small field of view wrist images than when larger fields of view are used (i.e., pelvis and hips). Uniform fat suppression technique is also more readily achieved with circumferential coils and the arm above the head so that the wrist is in the center of the magnet. Off-axis small field of view imaging (arm at the side) increases patient comfort and reduces motion artifact.[4] Metal artifacts from fixation devices may also cause image distortion. Proper planning of the examination, knowledge of suspected lesion location and positioning, pulse sequence and image plane orientation can reduce errors due to technical problems.[4]

Flow artifacts vary with different pulse sequences (Fig. 3-1) but are more of a problem in the peripheral extremity. When these artifacts enter the area of interest, the lesion can be obscured. In this setting, the images can be repeated following a change in the phase direction, which directs the flow artifact to go in the new phase plane and provides better visualization of the area of interest. Flow suppression techniques are also useful in reducing artifacts.[4]

The "magic angle" phenomenon may cause increased signal intensity in tendons or ligaments oriented 45° to 65° to the magnetic field (Bo).[6] The magnetic field (Bo) varies with the type of magnet. It is aligned along the bore of closed high-field systems, vertical on open magnets, and left to right in small-extremity units (Fig. 3-2). Confusion may be exaggerated in the hand and wrist where ligament and tendon orientation can be difficult to confirm on axial images. Proper positioning, use or radial or ulnar deviation and comparison with coronal or sagittal images will help prevent interpretation errors due to the magic angle phenomenon.[4,6]

This phenomenon occurs with short TE spin echo and many gradient echo sequences, but is not a problem with long TE or T2-weighted sequences.[1,4,6] Abnormal signal intensity that is not a magic angle phenomenon has also been described in the extensor carpi ulnaris tendon.[25] However, pathology is unlikely in the absence of tendon enlargement or fluid in the tendon sheath.[1]

Anatomic variants are important and should be recognized. These may include both soft-tissue (muscle, tendon, ligament, neural, and vascular) and osseous structures.[5,10,24,25]

OSSEOUS VARIANTS

The carpal bones develop from a single ossification center. Therefore, in general, conditions such as bipartite or tripartite carpal bones are uncommon.[8,13] Unfortunately, when these anomalies do occur, they usually involve the carpal bone most commonly fractured, the scaphoid.[13,17,18] The most common appearance is two separate scaphoid ossicles separated at the waist, a common sight for scaphoid fractures (Fig. 3-3D).[4,13,20] The capitate and hook of the hamate may also develop from multiple ossification centers. When this occurs, differentiation from fracture or fracture nonunion may be difficult on MR images.[4] Hypoplastic hamate hooks have also been described in female patients.[14,20]

Osseous coalitions may be fibrous, cartilaginous, or osseous.[27] The most common is lunotriquetral, but coalition between the capitate and hamate occurs in rare cases.[13,20,27] Idiopathic coalitions are more common in female and African-American individuals, occurring in up to 6% of the black population.[13,18] Lunotriquetral coalitions have been classified by Minaar (Fig. 3-3).[18] Type I coalitions are fibrous or cartilaginous and may be painful (Figs. 3-3A and 3-4). Type II coalitions are incomplete osseous fusions with a distal notch (Fig. 3-3B), and type III coalitions show complete osseous fusion (Figs. 3-3C and 3-5). Type IV coalitions (Fig. 3-3D) are complete osseous fusions with other carpal anomalies.[18,20,27]

Lunate articular variations may also occur. A type I lunate (Fig. 3-6A) has a single distal facet whereas a type II lunate (Fig. 3-6B) has a second small medial facet that articulates with the hamate. Both occur with about the same frequency.[27] Type II configuration is more often associated with degenerative arthritis and ulnar wrist

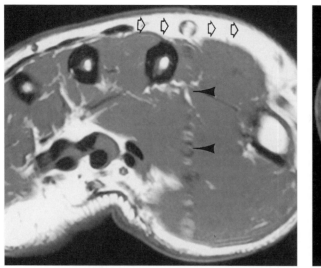
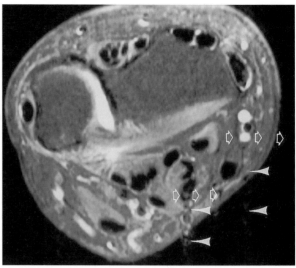

A   B

FIGURE 3-1. Axial T1-weighted image of the hand **(A)** and fat-suppressed T1-weighted arthrographic image of the wrist **(B)** demonstrating flow artifacts *(arrowheads)*. Swapping the phase direction would change the plane of the artifact *(open arrows)*.

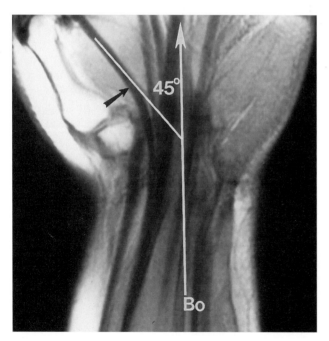

FIGURE 3-2. Coronal T1-weighted image of the tendons. Magic angle phenomenon could cause confusion with increased signal in the flexor pollicis longus tendon *(arrow)*, which is oriented 45° to the magnetic field (Bo).

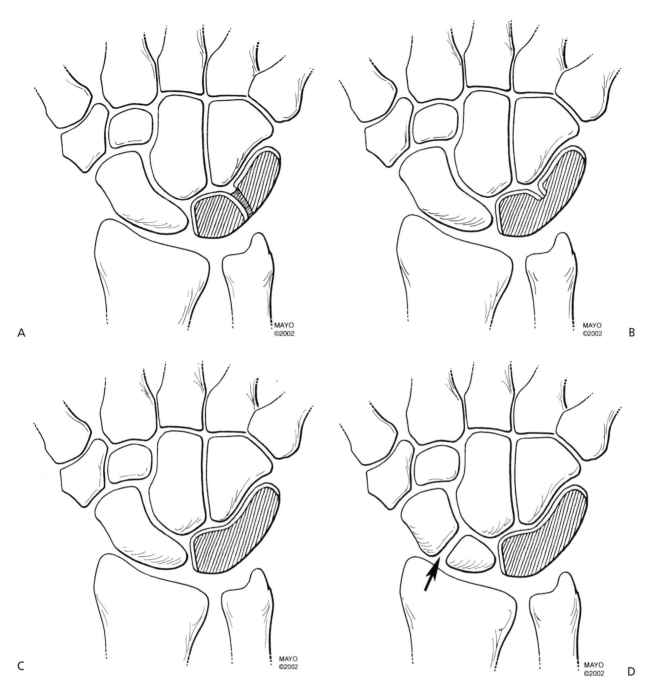

FIGURE 3-3. Lunotriquetral coalitions. **A:** Type I—fibrous or cartilaginous coalition. **B:** Type II—incomplete osseous fusion with a distal notch. **C:** Type III—complete osseous fusion. **D:** Type IV—complete osseous fusion with other carpal anomalies. In this case, a bipartite scaphoid *(arrow).*

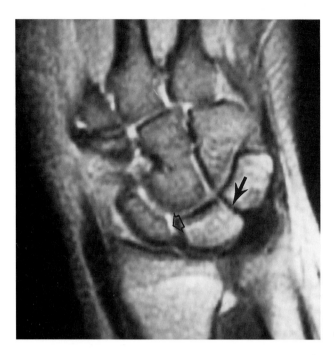

FIGURE 3-4. Coronal T2-weighted image demonstrating a fibrous (type I) lunotriquetral coalition *(arrow)*. Note the decreased space and low signal intensity. There is high signal intensity fluid between the scaphoid and lunate *(open arrow)*.

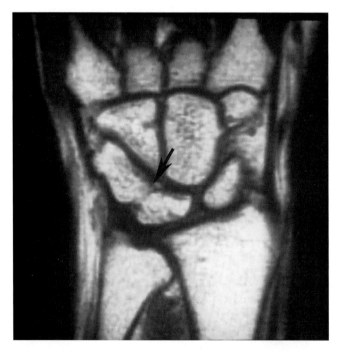

FIGURE 3-5. Coronal T1-weighted image demonstrates complete osseous (type III) fusion *(arrow)*.

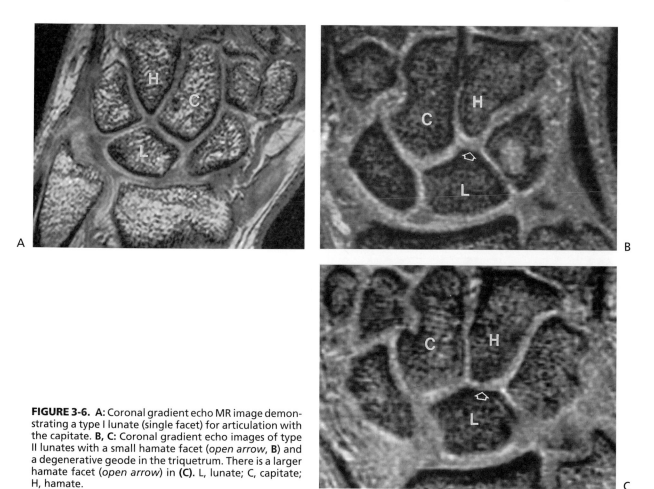

A

B

C

FIGURE 3-6. **A:** Coronal gradient echo MR image demonstrating a type I lunate (single facet) for articulation with the capitate. **B, C:** Coronal gradient echo images of type II lunates with a small hamate facet (*open arrow*, **B**) and a degenerative geode in the triquetrum. There is a larger hamate facet (*open arrow*) in (**C**). L, lunate; C, capitate; H, hamate.

pain.[19,27] Morphologic changes (types I and II) and secondary arthrosis are more easily appreciated on coronal MR images.[4]

An additional lunate variant may be seen on sagittal MR images. Nutrient vessels and ligament attachments (radiolunotriquetral and short radiolunate ligaments) may create an irregular appearance on the distal volar aspect of the lunate (Fig. 3-7).[10]

Small low signal intensity regions may be seen on coronal T1-weighted images. These represent vascular entry points or small bone islands and should not be confused with erosions (Fig. 3-8). If vascular, they may be high signal intensity on T2-weighted or contrast-enhanced images. Erosions are usually larger and more irregular.[20]

Subluxation of the distal radioulnar joint is most accurately assessed with axial images in supination, neutral, and pronated positions. During conventional MR studies, the wrist is pronated. In this position the ulna can look dorsally subluxed on axial and sagittal images (Fig. 3-9).[4,27]

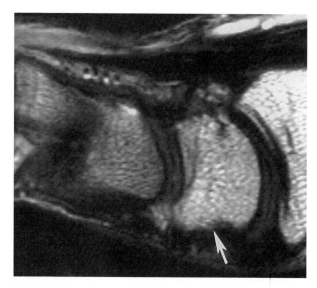

FIGURE 3-7. Sagittal T1-weighted MR image demonstrating volar irregularity (*arrow*) of the lunate due to ligament insertions.

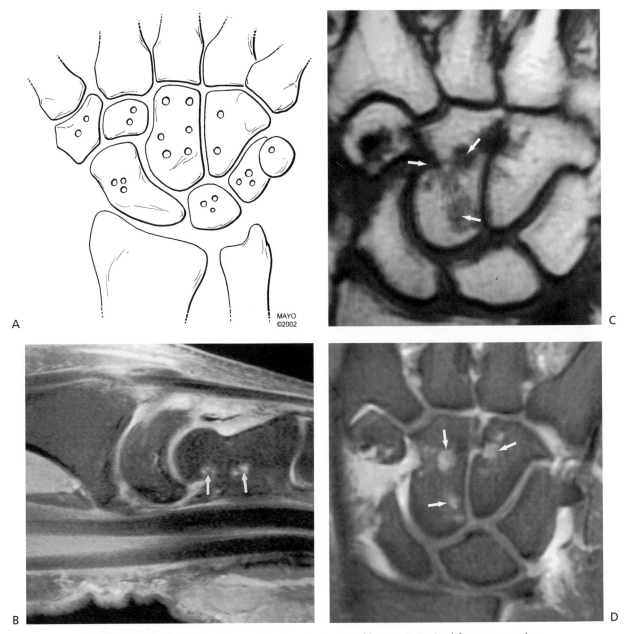

FIGURE 3-8. A: Illustration of vascular entry sites in carpal bones. **B:** Sagittal fat-suppressed enhanced image demonstrating two vascular entry sites *(arrows)* in the capitate. **C, D:** Coronal T1-weighted **(C)** and T2-weighted **(D)** MR images in a patient with rheumatoid arthritis and multiple carpal erosions *(arrows)*.

There are numerous ossicles in the hand and wrist (Fig. 3-10). Common ossicles and their location may be most easily appreciated on routine radiographs (Fig. 3-11).[4,13] They should not be confused with loose bodies or fracture fragments.

The lunula (Table 3-1) is an ossification center that lies between the triangular fibrocartilage (TFC) and the triquetrum. In some cases, it may fuse to the ulnar styloid (Fig. 3-12).[13]

The os styloideum, also known as the carpal boss, lies dorsal to the second and third metacarpal bases. This ossicle may be congenital or degenerative and may mimic a ganglion clinically (Fig. 3-10).[13,27]

The os triangulare (Table 3-1) is congenital and lies distal to the ulnar fovea.[13] The trapezium secondarium lies at the super medial border of the trapezium (Table 3-1, Fig. 3-10).[13,27] The epilunate lies dorsal to the lunate (Fig. 3-10) and because of its location may be easily mistaken for a loose body.[25] The os hamuli (Fig. 3-11) lies at the tip of the hamate hook (Table 3-1).[13] The os Gruber (Fig. 3-10) is uncommon but lies between the capitate, hamate, and third and fourth metacarpal bases.[9]

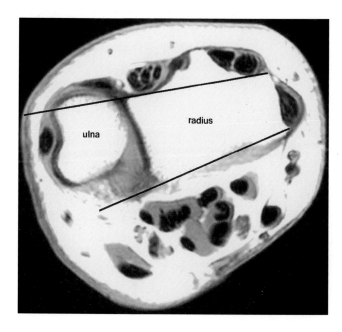

FIGURE 3-9. Axial T1-weighted MR image in the prone position. The ulna appears dorsally subluxed *(dark lines)*.

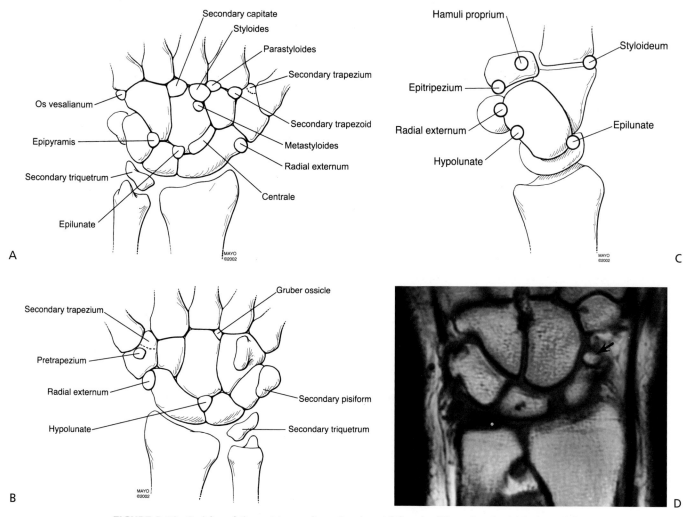

FIGURE 3-10. Ossicles of the wrist seen from the dorsal **(A)**, volar **(B)**, and sagittal **(C)** views. **(D)** Coronal T1-weighted MR image of an os centrale *(arrow)*.

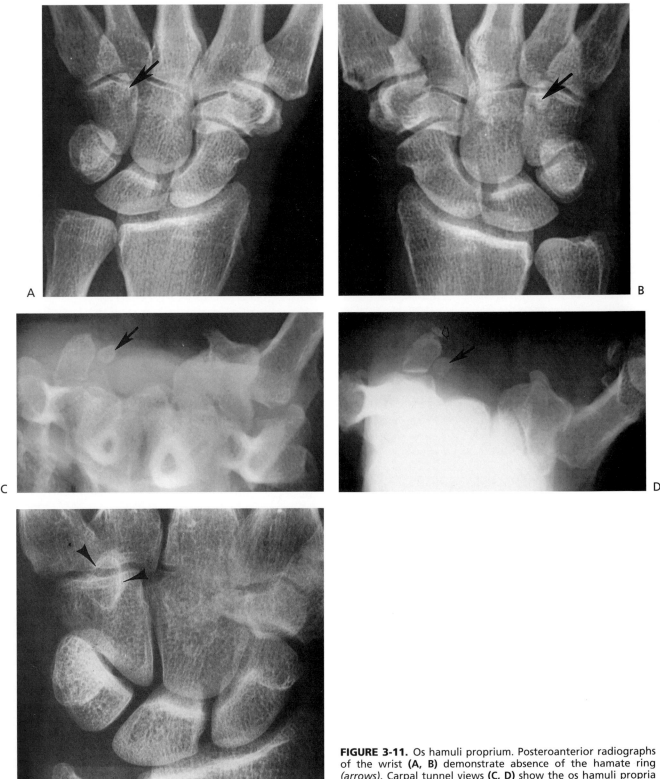

FIGURE 3-11. Os hamuli proprium. Posteroanterior radiographs of the wrist **(A, B)** demonstrate absence of the hamate ring *(arrows)*. Carpal tunnel views **(C, D)** show the os hamuli propria *(arrows)* and a small bipartite pisiform *(open arrow)*. **(E)** PA radiograph demonstrating the normal hamate ring *(arrowheads)* for comparison.

TABLE 3-1. COMMON OSSICLES OF THE HAND AND WRIST[9,13,20,27]

Ossicle	Location
Lunula	Between TFC Complex and triquetrum may fuse to ulnar styloid
Os styloideum	Dorsal to 2nd and 3rd metacarpal bases
Os triangulare	Distal to ulnar fovea
Trapezium secondarium	Superomedial aspect of trapezium
Epilunate	Dorsal to lunate
Os hamuli	Adjacent to hamate hook
Os Gruber	Between capitate, hamate and 3rd and 4th metacarpal bases

TFC, triangular fibrocartilage.

SOFT-TISSUE VARIANTS

Numerous muscle/tendon anomalies have been described in the hand and wrist. The anomalies may mimic soft-tissue masses or result in neurovascular compression.[5,7,21,22,27,28]

The accessory abductor digiti minimi (Fig. 3-13) is a common variant reported in 24% of patients. The muscle may take its origin from several locations including the palmar carpal ligament, the palmaris longus tendon, and the fascia of the forearm. It inserts along with the abductor digiti minimi on the medial aspect of the fifth proximal phalanx (Fig. 3-13).[26,29] Ulnar or median nerve symptoms may be associated with this anomaly.[22,26]

The extensor digitorum brevis manus muscle (Fig. 3-14) is reported in 1% to 3% of the general population.[5,25] The muscle originates on the distal radius or dorsal radiocarpal ligament and inserts on the distal second metacarpal. This anomalous muscle is generally asymptomatic but can present with tenderness and mimic a ganglion.[5]

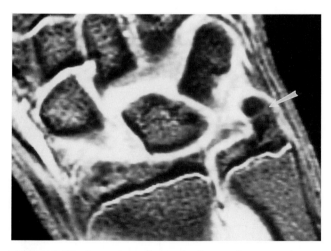

FIGURE 3-12. Coronal gradient echo image demonstrating an elongated ulnar styloid with a faint intermediate signal intensity line *(arrow)* due to a partially fused lunula.

The lumbrical muscles normally originate from the flexor digitorum longus tendons distal to the carpal tunnel. In 22% of patients the origin is more proximally in the carpal tunnel. When the fingers are flexed, the contracted muscles can cause carpal tunnel symptoms.[14,26] This anomalous origin may also mimic a soft-tissue mass or synovitis.[5,17]

The palmaris longus (Fig. 3-15) typically takes its origin with the other flexors on the medial epicondyle.[15] Typically there is a short belly with the tendon inserting on the palmar aponeurosis of the hand (Fig. 3-15A).[15,23] In up to 13% of patients the muscle is absent.[26] There are numerous variations including the palmaris longus inversus where the muscle belly is located distally instead of proximally (Fig. 3-15B). This variant is more common in females and can cause exercise-induced median nerve compression.[23] Other variants include the nontendinous variant, central tendon with muscle bellies proximally and distally, and a bifid muscle with two distal tendon insertions. Variants may mimic soft-tissue masses or cause nerve compression (Fig. 3-15E).[15,23,26]

Anomalies of the flexor digitorum superficialis may result in a distal muscle belly along the proximal phalanx. This anomalie may mimic a soft-tissue mass.[26,29] An anomalous origin of the flexor digiti minimi may compress the ulnar nerve.[20]

An accessory extensor pollicis longus tendon has also been described in the third dorsal compartment. The patient presented with pain and tenderness relieved by excision of the accessory muscle.[3,25]

Variations in the ligaments and TFC complex may also cause errors in image interpretation.[2,4,11,24,25] The TFC attaches to the ulnar styloid–fovea junction, which contains a rich vascular supply and fibrofatty tissue that may cause confusion due to the intermediate signal intensity in this region on T1- and T2-weighted sequences (Fig. 3-16). The radial attachment of the TFC inserts on hyalin cartilage and not cortical bone. This results in a focal area of intermediate signal intensity between the low-signal TFC and radial cortical bone (Fig. 3-16B).[25] Intermediate signal intensity may be seen near the ulnar attachment. Degeneration in the TFC may also cause intermediate signal intensity similar to the changes seen in the meniscus of the knee (Fig. 3-16).[4,25] True tears in the TFC have high (fluid) signal intensity compared with the intermediate signal intensity seen due to the anatomic structures at the TFC attachments.[4,25]

Variations in the appearance of the scapholunate, lunotriquetral, and other supporting ligaments of the wrist have also been described.[4,25] These changes will be discussed in Chapter 4.

Variations in the median nerve may also cause confusion. Though carpal tunnel syndrome is a clinical diagnosis, MRI is useful for anatomic evaluation. Adjacent pathology is also easily detected. The normal median nerve is elliptical with variable signal intensity. Signal intensity may be similar to that of muscle or fat on T1- and T2-weighted sequences.[12,25]

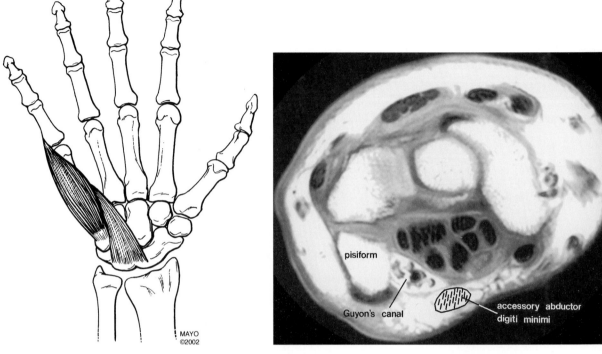

FIGURE 3-13. Accessory abductor digiti minimi. **A:** Illustration showing the accessory abductor digiti minimi with an oblique course from palmar carpal ligaments to insert along with the abductor digiti minimi on the medial fifth proximal phalanx. **B:** Axial MR image demonstrating the location of the muscle and relationship to ulnar nerve and Guyon's canal. Normally there is no muscle in this region at the pisiform level.

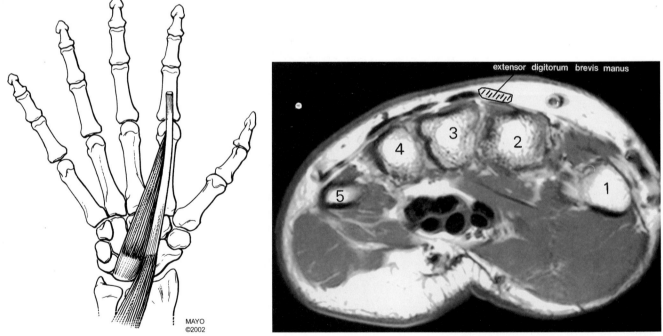

FIGURE 3-14. Extensor digitorum manus muscle. **A:** Illustration of the extensor digitorum brevis manus medial to the extensor tendon of the index finger. The muscle arises from the dorsal carpal ligament and inserts on the second metacarpal. **B:** Axial MR image demonstrating the location of the extensor digitorum brevis manus muscle at the level of the metacarpal bases. The muscle is radial to the extensor tendons between the second and third metacarpals.

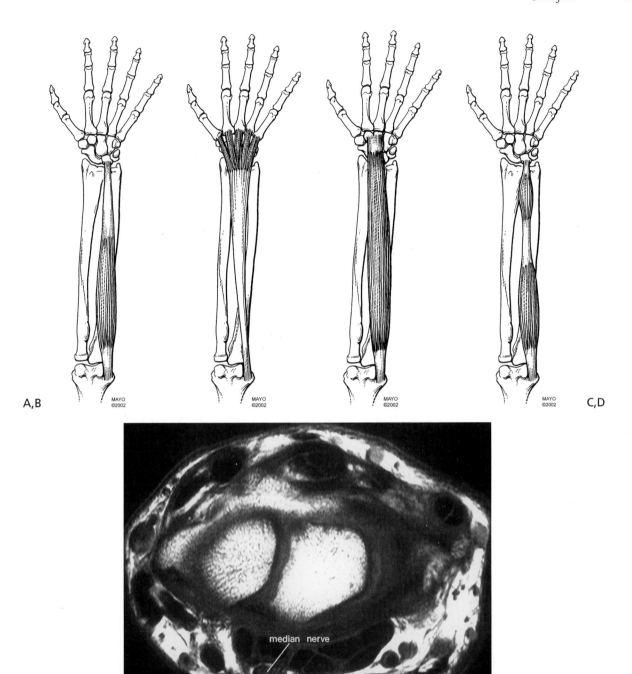

A,B

C,D

E

FIGURE 3-15. Palmaris longus muscle. Illustrations of the normal **(A)**, inverse variant **(B)**, total muscle variant **(C)**, and proximal and distal muscle bellies **(D)**. Axial MR image **(E)** demonstrating the location of palmaris longus inversus (distal muscle belly) variant at the level of the radiocarpal joint. Note the relationship to the median nerve.

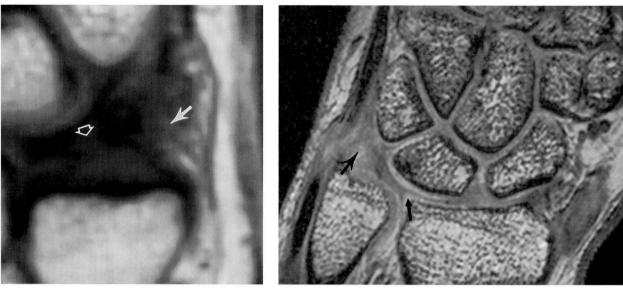

A

B

FIGURE 3-16. A: Coronal T1-weighted image of the triangular fibrocartilage with intermediate signal intensity near the ulnar attachment *(arrow)* and in its central portion *(open arrow)*. This is not a tear. **B:** Coronal gradient echo image demonstrating normal intermediate signal near the ulnar attachment *(arrow)* and at the cartilage attachment to the radius *(small arrow)*.

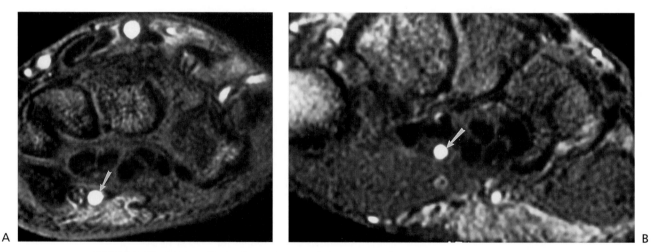

A

B

FIGURE 3-17. Axial gradient echo MR images of aberrant vessels. **A:** Aberrant radial artery *(arrow)* near the ulnar nerve in Guyon's canal. **B:** Aberrant vessels with the larger branch *(arrow)* adjacent to the median nerve.

Therefore, the signal intensity should not be considered abnormal unless it is increased or greater than that of fat on T2-weighted sequences.[25]

A bifid median nerve has been described in 2.8% of the population. A persistent median artery may be present between the nerve segments.[16]

Vascular anomalies (Fig. 3-17) are also common. Typically, they are not symptomatic unless located adjacent to neural structures.[4]

REFERENCES

1. Anderson MW, Benedetti P, Walter J, et al. MR appearance of the extensor digitorum manus brevis muscle: a pseudo tumor of the hand. AJR 1995;164:1477–1479.
2. Anderson MW, Kaplan PA, Dussault RG, et al. Magnetic resonance imaging of the wrist. Curr Probl Diagn Radiol 1998; Nov–Dec:191–219.
3. Beatty JD, Remedios D, McCullough CJ. An accessory extensor tendon of the thumb as a cause of dorsal wrist pain. J Hand Surg 2000;25B:110–111.
4. Berquist TH. MRI of the musculoskeletal system, 4th ed. Philadelphia: Lippincott Williams & Wilkins, 2001:773–841.
5. Capelastegui A, Astigarraga E, Fernandez-Canton G, et al. Masses and pseudo masses of the hand and wrist: MR findings in 134 cases. Skel Radiol 1999;28:498–507.
6. Erickson SJ, Cox IH, Hyde JS, et al. Effect of tendon orientation on MR signal intensity: a manifestation of the magic angle effect. Radiology 1991;181:389–392.
7. Fakih RR, Thomas R, Mansour A. The extensor brevis manus. Bull Hosp Joint Dis 1997;56:115–116.
8. Kauer JMG. The mechanism of the carpal joint. Clin Orthop 1986;202:16–26.
9. Köse N, Özcelik A, Günal I. The crowded wrist: a case with accessory carpal bones. Acta Orthop Scand 1999;70:96–98.
10. Lichtman DM. The wrist and its disorders. Philadelphia: WB Saunders, 1988.
11. Metz VM, Schatter M, Dock WI, et al. Age associated changes of the triangular fibrocartilage of the wrist: evaluation of diagnostic performance of MR imaging. Radiology 1992;184:217–220.
12. Middleton WD, Kneeland JB, Kellman GM, et al. MR imaging of the carpal tunnel: normal anatomy and preliminary findings in carpal tunnel syndrome. AJR 1987;148:307–316.
13. O'Rahilly R. A survey of carpal and tarsal anomalies. J Bone Joint Surg 1953;35A:626–641.
14. Pierre-Jerome C, Bekkelund SI, Husby G, et al. MRI anatomic variants of the wrist in women. Surg Radiol Anat 1996;18:37–41.
15. Polesuk BS, Helms CA. Hypertrophied palmaris longus muscle, a pseudo mass of the forearm: MR appearance. Case report and a review of the literature. Radiology 1998;207:361–362.
16. Propeck T, Quinn TJ, Jacobson JA, et al. Sonography and MR imaging of bifid median nerve and anatomic and histologic correlation. AJR 2000;175:1721–1725.
17. Rosse C, Rosse PC. Hollingshead's textbook of anatomy. Philadelphia: Lippincott–Raven Publishers, 1997.
18. Simmons BP, McKenzie WD. Symptomatic carpal coalition. J Hand Surg 1985;10A:190–193.
19. Sagerman SD, Hauck RM, Palmer AK. Lunate morphology: can it be predicted on routine radiographs? J Hand Surg 1995;20A:38–41.
20. Schmidt H, Freyschmidt J. Kohler/Zimmer's borderlands of normal and early pathologic findings in skeletal radiology, 4th ed. New York: Thieme Medical Publishers, 1993.
21. Spinner RJ, Lui RE, Spinver M. Compression of the medial half of the deep branch of the ulnar nerve by anomalous origin of the flexor digiti minimi. J Bone Joint Surg 1996;78A:427–430.
22. Still JM, Kleinert HE. Anomalous muscles and nerve entrapment in the wrist and hand. Plast Reconstr Surg 1973;52:394–400.
23. Schuurman AH, Van Gils APG. Reversed palmaris longus muscle on MRI: report of four cases. Eur Radiol 2000;10:1242–1244.
24. Timins ME, Johnke JP, Krah SE, et al. MR imaging of major carpal stabilizing ligaments: normal anatomy and clinical examples. Radiographics 1995;14:575–587.
25. Timins ME, O'Connell SE, Erickson SE, et al. MR imaging of the wrist: normal findings that may simulate disease. Radiographics 1996;16:987–995.
26. Timins ME. Muscular anatomic variants of the wrist and hand: findings on MR imaging. AJR 1999;172:1397–1401.
27. Timins ME. Osseous anatomic variants of the wrist: findings on MR imaging. AJR 1999;173:339–344.
28. Zeiss J, Jakab E. MR demonstration of an anomalous muscle in a patient with coexistent carpal and ulnar tunnel syndrome: case report and literature summary. Clin Imaging 1995;19:102–105.
29. Zeiss J, Guilliam-Haidet L. MR demonstration of anomalous muscles about the volar aspect of the wrist and forearm. Clin Imaging 1996;20:219–221.

4

TRAUMA

THOMAS H. BERQUIST
JEFFREY JAMES PETERSON
LAURA WASYLENKO BANCROFT
KIMBERLY K. AMRAMI

Magnetic resonance imaging (MRI) techniques in conjunction with other imaging studies provides useful information for acute and chronic osseous and soft-tissue injuries of the hand and wrist.[10,11,22,70,86,87,90] Selection of the proper imaging techniques and MR approach requires a thorough knowledge of anatomy and the suspected injury. This makes communication with the referring physician essential to provide the necessary information and, optimally, define the extent and type of injury.[10,11]

OSSEOUS INJURIES

Most suspected osseous injuries are initially imaged with routine radiography or computed radiography. Subtle and complex injuries may require additional studies such as computed tomography (CT) or MRI for detection and complete evaluation.[10,11,27,58] Osseous injuries (Table 4-1) include complete fractures, incomplete fractures, physeal injury or fracture, stress fractures, and bone bruises.[4,10,36,47,52]

It is important to detect fractures early, especially scaphoid fractures, so as to reduce morbidity and avoid complications. MRI is suggested when radiographs are negative but clinical findings suggest an osseous injury or when healing does not occur in the expected time. Up to 35% of fractures identified by MRI cannot be detected on radiographs.[52]

Distal Radius and Ulna Fractures

Fractures of the distal radius and ulna are common and are usually easily identified on radiographs or computer radiographic images.[10,11] Physeal injuries may be subtle, requiring MRI for detection (Fig. 4-1).[4,29] In children, 40% of physeal injuries involve the distal radius and ulnar physeal injuries account for 5% of physeal fractures.[7] Included in the spectrum of gymnast's wrist are physeal injuries as well as soft-tissue injuries, which will be discussed later in this chapter.[21,31] High loads applied to the wrist during gymnastics most commonly

result in injuries when athletes are 12 to 14 years of age and practice more than 20 hours per week.[10,21] Evaluation of physeal fracture complications is also easily accomplished with MRI.[10,11,20]

Radiographs may demonstrate physeal irregularity, especially involving the volar aspect of the radius (Fig. 4-2). Cystic metaphyseal changes may also be evident.[21,31] Ulnar positive variance has been described with this condition. Patients with stage I gymnast's wrist have clinical symptoms with no radiographic features. Stage II disease includes clinical features with physeal irregularity (Fig. 4-2). Stage III disease includes features of stage II plus ulnar positive variance.[21,31]

Carpal Fractures

Carpal fractures are rare in children but common in adults.[7,19] Scaphoid fractures occur most commonly in adults and children. However, in children scaphoid fractures account for only 2.9% of hand and waist fractures. In adults fractures most often involve the wrist, whereas in children the distal third is most commonly involved.[7,10,56] Fractures of the triquetrum are the second most common carpal fracture followed by the capitate and lunate.[7,10]

Carpal fractures may be very subtle. Early detection is important to reduce morbidity and complications.[27,59] Up to 35% of subtle fractures are overlooked on initial radiographs.[42,52] Computed tomography and radionuclide studies are important for detection of early subtle lesions.[4] However, MRI is sensitive and specific for subtle fractures, including bone bruises.[10,66,76]

The MRI approach varies depending on the suspected fracture.[11,13,14] Marrow edema is low intensity on T1- and high intensity on T2-weighted images.[10,11,36,66,76] The fracture line is typically low intensity on both sequences when there is trabecular compression (Figs. 4-3 and 4-4). Increased signal intensity is seen on T2-weighted sequences when fragments are separated.[10,11] Image planes (Fig. 4-5) are important to consider for complete evaluation, especially

**TABLE 4-1. FRACTURES OF THE HAND AND
WRIST**[4,10,27,47]

Complete
Incomplete one cortex
Bone bruise
Osteochondral
Stress fractures
Physeal fractures

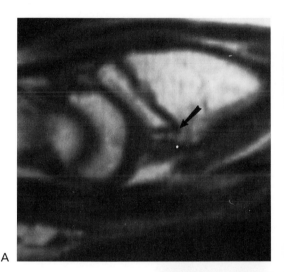

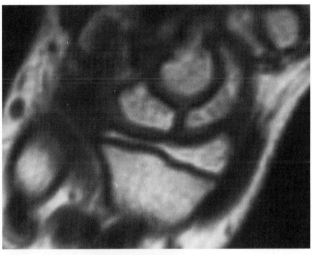

FIGURE 4-1. Old radial physeal fracture with a bony bar involving the volar 10% of the radial growth plate. T1-weighted MR images in the sagittal **(A)**, coronal **(B)**, and axial **(C)** planes demonstrate the extent of the bar *(arrows)* allowing preoperative planning for resection. T2-weighted sequences are preferred in most cases.

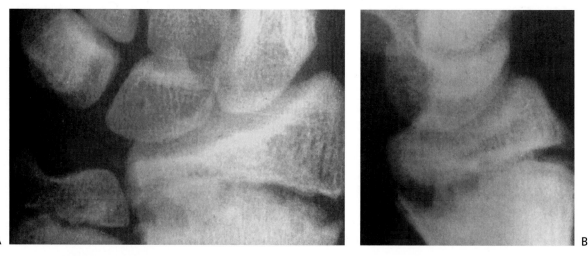

FIGURE 4-2. Posteroanterior **(A)** and lateral **(B)** radiographs demonstrate irregularity of the radial growth plate due to gymnast's wrist.

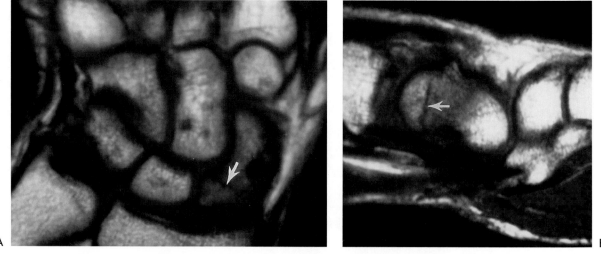

FIGURE 4-3. Coronal **(A)** and sagittal **(B)** T1-weighted images demonstrate an undisplaced scaphoid fracture *(arrow)*. Note the normal fragment position on the sagittal image **(B)**.

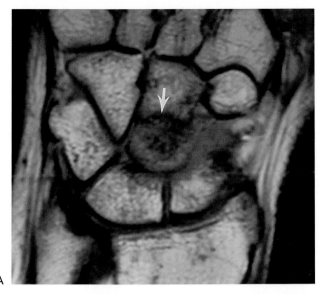 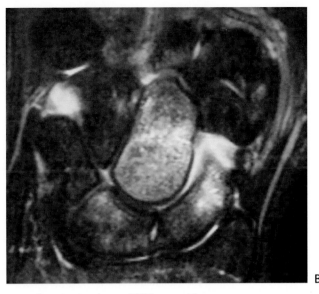

FIGURE 4-4. Coronal T1-weighted **(A)** and fat-suppressed contrast-enhanced **(B)** images. The capitate fracture *(arrow)* is clearly seen on the T1-weighted image **(A)**. There is edema in the fracture line and marrow on the postcontrast image **(B)**.

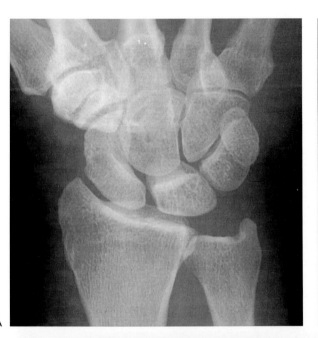 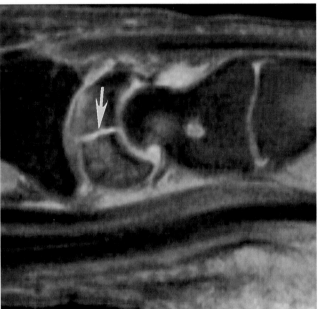

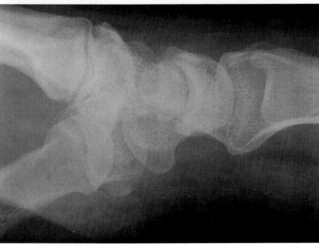

FIGURE 4-5. Posteroanterior **(A)** and lateral **(B)** radiographs of the wrist do not identify a fracture. Sagittal contrast-enhanced fat-suppressed T1-weighted image **(C)** clearly demonstrates the transverse lunate fracture *(arrow)*.

TABLE 4-2. CARPAL FRACTURE: IMAGE PLANES

Osseous Structure	Image Planes
Scaphoid	Coronal, oblique sagittal
Lunate	Coronal, sagittal
Triquetrum	Coronal, axial or oblique sagittal
Pisiform	Axial, sagittal
Trapezium	Coronal, axial
Trapezoid	Coronal, axial
Capitate	Coronal, sagittal
Hamate	Coronal, axial[a]

[a]Best for hamate hook.

of scaphoid fractures (Table 4-2).[55] Sagittal images of the scaphoid in the plane of the structure (oblique sagittal) are essential to evaluate deformity.[10]

Most carpal fractures are easily detected on MR images. Subtle dorsal triquetral fractures can be overlooked.[52]

Metacarpal/Phalangeal Fractures

Metacarpal and phalangeal fractures usually are obvious on routine radiographs. Therefore, other imaging studies, including MRI, are rarely indicated. Subtle fractures, associated soft-tissue injury, and complications can be evaluated with MRI. Axial and sagittal or coronal T1- and T2-weighted sequences are most useful (Fig. 4-6). Coronal or three-dimensional gradient echo images may be required when ligament or capsular injury is suspected.[10,11]

Fracture Complications

Complications associated with osseous injury vary with patient age and site of injury. In children or the immature skeleton, physeal injuries can result in articular deformity due to premature growth plate closure or overgrowth (Fig. 4-1).[4,10] Other complications include delayed union,

malunion, nonunion, and avascular necrosis and soft-tissue injuries.

Physeal injuries may result in fibrous or osseous bars leading to asymmetry of the joint surface. This can be easily evaluated with MRI when surgical resection is considered.[11,25] Three-dimensional gradient echo or oblique image planes to optimize growth plate evaluation can determine the extent of the bar and whether resection is an option. Use of T1- and T2-weighted or gradient echo sequences allows differentiation of fibrous, cartilaginous, and osseous bars (Fig. 4-1).[10,25,29]

In a similar fashion, MRI can be used to evaluate fibrous union and nonunion using T1- and T2-weighted sequences (Fig. 4-7). Use of the appropriate image planes (Table 4-2) is especially important when evaluating the scaphoid for fracture union and "hump-back" deformities (Fig. 4-8).[10,42]

Gadolinium-enhanced fat-suppressed T1-weighted images are useful to evaluate avascular necrosis and nonunion.[11,13] Avascular necrosis occurs in up to 30% of proximal scaphoid fractures (Fig. 4-9).[70]

Magnetic resonance imaging can also be used to detect soft-tissue injury or complications associated with fractures. These may include ligament, tendon, and neurovascular injury or soft-tissue interposition (Fig. 4-10).

SOFT-TISSUE INJURIES

Soft-tissue injuries to the hand and wrist may result from acute trauma, recurrent microtrauma with degeneration, or overuse syndromes.[4,8,10,11,22,76] Routine radiographs are useful as a screening tool to exclude associated osseous injury, malunion, nonunion, or other subtle changes that may suggest the associated soft-tissue injury.[10,70,76] Depending on clinical evaluation and radiographic findings, ultrasound, CT, MRI, or conventional or MR arthrography (MRA) may be the next examination selected.[3,10,68]

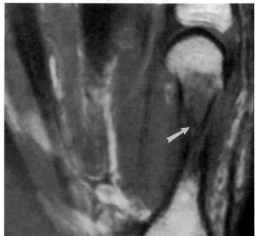

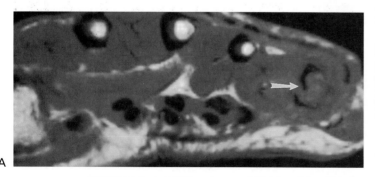

A   B

FIGURE 4-6. Axial **(A)** and coronal **(B)** T1-weighted images of an unsuspected metacarpal fracture *(arrow)* with adjacent low signal intensity edema.

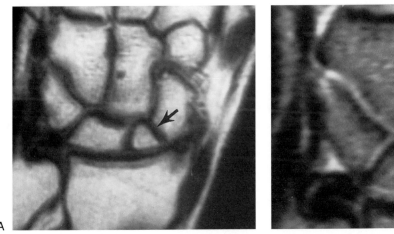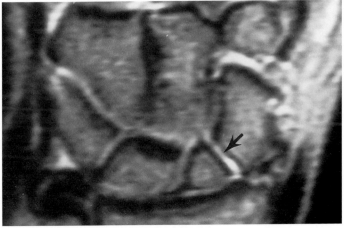

A B

FIGURE 4-7. Coronal T1- **(A)** and T2-weighted **(B)** images show low signal intensity in the fracture line **(A)** and sclerotic margins with fluid in the fracture line due to nonunion *(arrow)*.

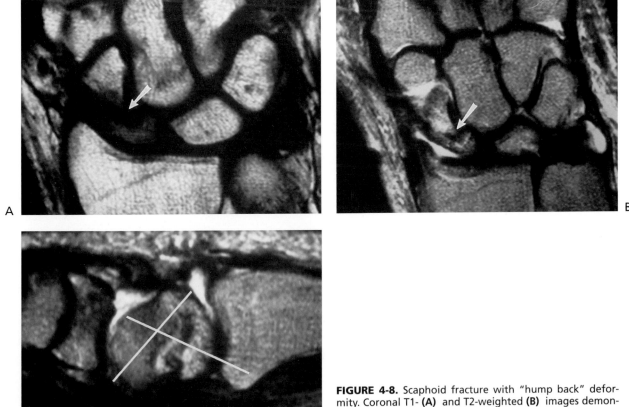

A B

C

FIGURE 4-8. Scaphoid fracture with "hump back" deformity. Coronal T1- **(A)** and T2-weighted **(B)** images demonstrate a displaced scaphoid fracture *(arrow)*. **(C)** Sagittal T2-weighted image demonstrates the angular (humpback) deformity (lines).

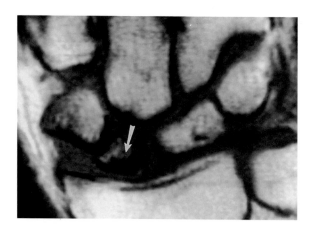

FIGURE 4-9. Coronal T1-weighted image of a proximal pole scaphoid fractures with low signal intensity in the proximal fragment *(arrow)* due to avascular necrosis.

Triangular Fibrocartilage Complex

The triangular fibrocartilage (TFC) complex includes the disc-supporting ligaments and extensor carpi ulnaris (ECU) tendon (see Chapter 1).[5,10,15,37,60]

Patients with injury to the TFC complex present with ulnar wrist pain. Associated ulnar styloid fracture and lunotriquetral ligament tears (70%) may be associated with TFC complex tears.[60,63,70] Traumatic tears are more common in younger patients and usually occur near the radial attach-

ment at the junction of the thicker vascular zone and thin avascular zone. Ulnar minus variance is commonly present in these patients.[22,70] Degenerative tears occur more commonly in the vascular zone near the ulnar attachment. These tears are more likely to heal without surgical intervention. Degenerative tears may be associated with ulnar positive variance and ulnar lunate impaction syndrome.[15,70]

The Palmer Classification is commonly used to define the type of TFC complex tear and associated findings (Fig. 4-11).[63] Type I tears are traumatic and type II tears degenerative

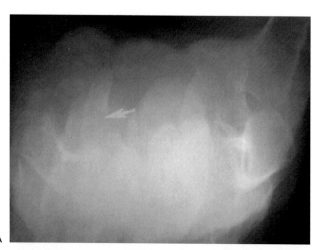

A

FIGURE 4-10. Carpal tunnel view **(A)** demonstrates a fracture of the hamate hook *(arrow).* Axial T1-weighted **(B)** and short TI inversion recovery (STIR) **(C)** images demonstrate the separated fragments *(arrowheads)* with the flexor tendon *(arrow)* between the fragments.

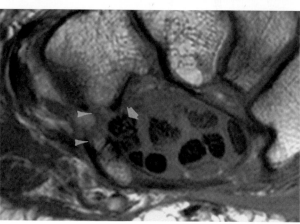

B

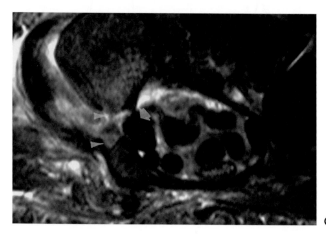

C

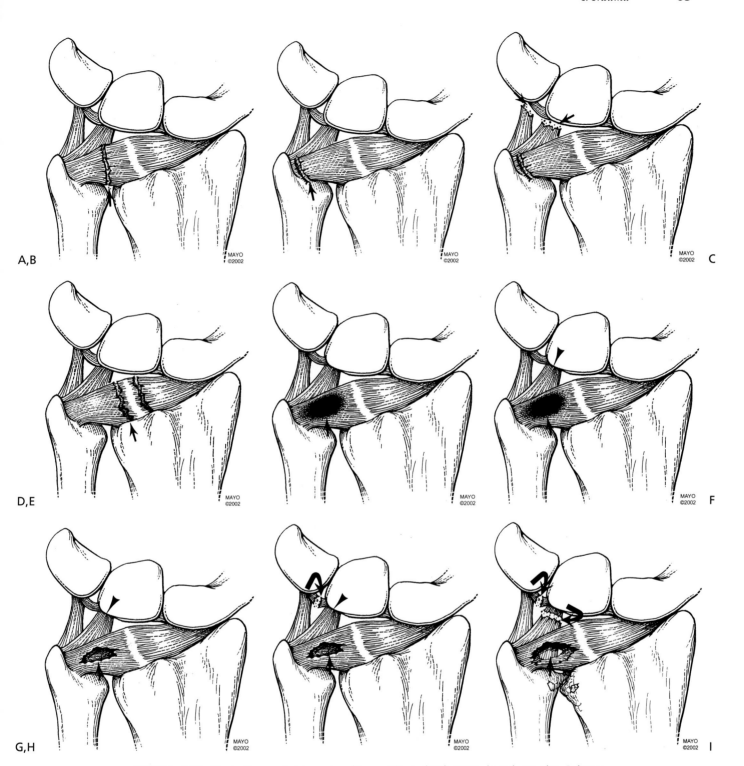

FIGURE 4-11. Illustrations of triangular fibrocartilage (TFC) tears based on the Palmer Classification.[63] **A:** Type IA: traumatic central perforation *(arrow)*. **B:** Type IB: ulnar avulsion *(arrow)* with or without distal ulnar fracture. **C:** Type IC: distal avulsion, with peripheral volar attachment tears of the ulnolunate and ulnotriquetral ligaments *(arrows)*. **D:** Type ID: radial avulsion *(arrow)* in sigmoid notch region, with or without radial fracture. **E:** Type IIA: degenerative TFC complex wear *(arrow)*. **F:** Type IIB: degenerative TFC wear *(arrow)* with lunate or ulnar chondromalacia *(arrowhead)*. **G:** Type IIC: TFC perforation *(arrow)* with lunate or ulnar chondromalacia *(arrowhead)*. **H:** Type IID: TFC perforation *(arrow)* with lunate or ulnar chondromalacia *(arrowhead)* and lunotriquetral ligament tear *(curved arrow)*. **I:** Type IIE: TFC perforation *(arrow)* with complex perforations *(curved arrows)* and ulnocarpal arthrosis *(open arrows)*.

TABLE 4-3. TRIANGULAR FIBROCARTILAGE COMPLEX TEARS, PALMER CLASSIFICATION[60,63]

Category	MRI Features	Comments
I. Traumatic		
A. Central perforation (Fig. 4-11A)	Linear increased signal intensity T2-weighted sequence 2–3 mm from radial attachment	Avascular portion, may not heal.
B. Ulnar avulsion (Fig. 4-11B)	Increased signal at ulnar attachment T2-weighted sequence	May have ulnar base fracture and dorsal and palmar radioulnar ligament tears. Vascular zone, so may heal.
C. Distal avulsion (Fig. 4-11C)	Increased signal at ulnar attachment and ulnolunate and ulnotriquetral ligament attachment on T2-weighted sequence	May lead to ulnar translation.
D. Radial avulsion (Fig. 4-11D)	Increased signal at radial attachment on T2-weighted sequence	May have associated radial fracture. Avascular so heals poorly.
II. Degenerative		
A. TFC central degeneration (Fig. 4-11E)	Intermediate signal PD and T2-weighted sequence	—
B. TFC degeneration with lunate chondromalacia (Fig. 4-11F)	Same as "A" with thinning or ↑ signal in lunate articular cartilage	—
C. TFC perforation and chondromalacia (Fig. 4-11 G)	Signal increases on T2-weighted second echo and lunate cartilage changes	—
D. TFC perforation, chondromalacia, and lunotriquetral tear (Fig. 4-11H)	Same as "C" plus linear ↑ signal in lunotriquetral ligament	—
E. Features of "D" plus ulnocarpal and radioulnar arthritis (Fig. 4-11I)	Same as "D" plus osteophytes and cartilage thinning in ulnocarpal and radioulnar joints	—

TFC, triangular fibrocartilage; PD, profondensity.

(Table 4-3).[60,63] Type IA and IB lesions are the most common traumatic injuries.[63] Degenerative lesions lead to initial degeneration of the TFC with progression to perforation (type IIC) and associated arthropathy (type IIE).[63]

The TFC complex may be evaluated indirectly based on radiographic features. Ulnar positive variance, radioulnar and ulnar lunate arthrosis, and changes in the ulnar styloid may be evident (Fig. 4-12).[10,60,70] Arthrography of the radiocarpal or distal radioulnar joints (DRUJs) is useful (Fig. 4-13). Keep in mind that asymptomatic perforations may be evident in 27% of middle-aged patients. Also, arthrography may be more accurate than MRI for associated lunotriquetral ligament tears.[44,60,70]

Both conventional and MR arthrography have been compared with surgery and arthroscopy for evaluating the TFC complex.[35,45,69,70,77,82,91] Evaluation with MRI can be accomplished using conventional spin echo T1- and T2-weighted (2000/20,80) sequences or T2* gradient echo

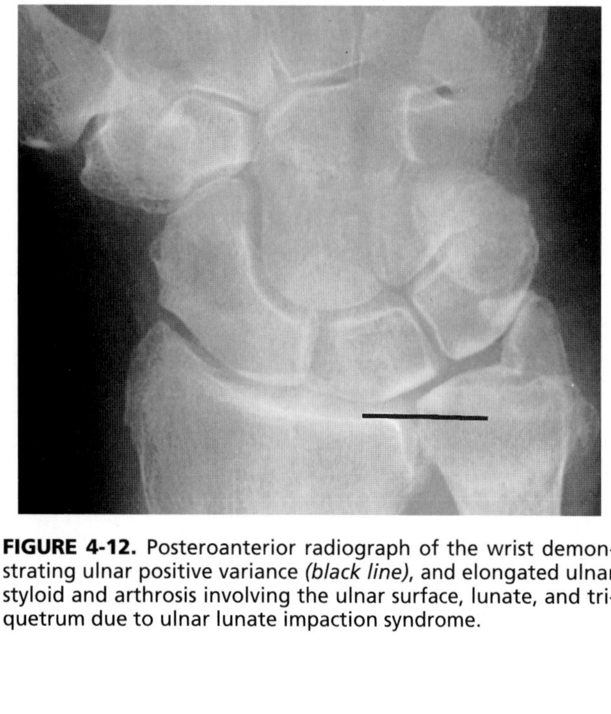

FIGURE 4-12. Posteroanterior radiograph of the wrist demonstrating ulnar positive variance *(black line)*, and elongated ulnar styloid and arthrosis involving the ulnar surface, lunate, and triquetrum due to ulnar lunate impaction syndrome.

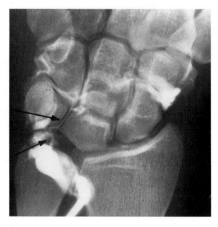

FIGURE 4-13. Distal radioulnar joint arthrogram shows contrast flowing through a triangular fibrocartilage tear (1) and lunotriquetral ligament tear (2) into the intercarpal joint.

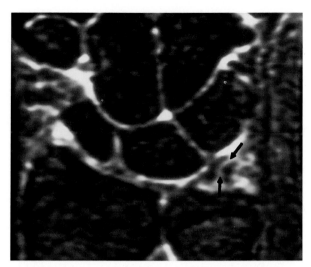

FIGURE 4-14. Coronal gradient echo image demonstrating a complete *(arrows)* central triangular fibrocartilage tear.

sequences (Fig. 4-14).[11,58] Fat suppression is useful with T1-weighted and fast spin echo (FSE) T2-weighted sequences. The latter are less useful.[58] High-resolution three-dimensional gradient echo sequences (50/20, FA 20°) with a 9-cm field of view (FOV), 256 × 256 matrix, and 1-mm-thick sections have been reported to demonstrate TFC complex tears with a sensitivity of 100%, specificity of 53%, and accuracy of 79%.[45] The location of the defect is also significant. The sensitivity for central defects is 91%, radial defects 86% to 100%, and ulnar avulsions only 25% to 50%.[61]

In a recent study, Haims et al.[37] evaluated ulnar attachment tears. They compared indirect MRA and conventional MRI findings to surgical findings. The MRI sensitivity was 17%, specificity 79%, and accuracy 64%. Using high signal intensity on T2-weighted sequences as a marker, the sensitivity was 42%, specificity 63%, and accuracy only 55%. These findings, along with other reports, suggest that MRI is not adequate for the evaluation of peripheral tears (Fig. 4-15).[37,61] This finding is significant in that peripheral tears can be repaired (good vascularity) whereas central tears are typically debrided.[37]

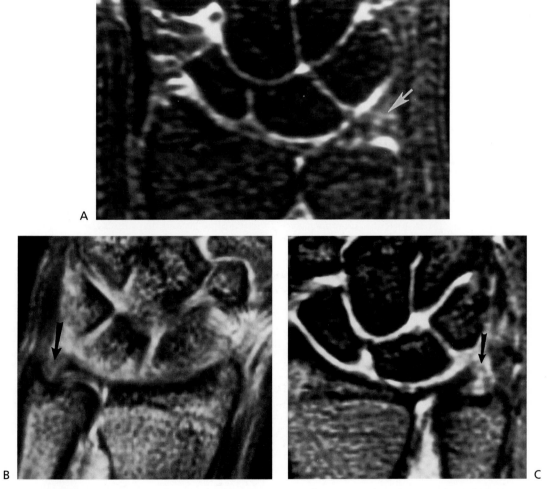

FIGURE 4-15. A: Coronal gradient echo image of normal triangular fibrocartilage *(arrow)*. **B, C:** Coronal gradient echo images with variable increased signal intensity peripherally *(arrow)*. No tears were present.

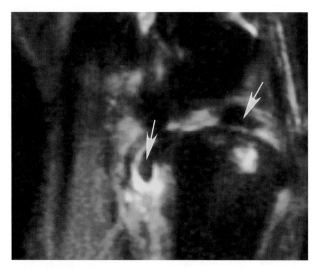

FIGURE 4-16. Sagittal fat suppressed arthrogram image demonstrating a central perforation with displaced fragments *(arrows)*.

When MRA was compared with conventional arthrography and arthroscopy, the sensitivity of MRA was 100%, specificity 90%, and accuracy 97%. Lesion localization was equally accurate (Figs. 4-16 and 4-17).[69] In some series, conventional wrist arthrography is as or more accurate for TFC tears, especially if lunotriquetral tears are also present (Fig. 4-13).[54,62,77]

There are multiple impaction syndromes that result in ulnar-sided wrist pain. Certain syndromes are associated with TFC defects. Table 4-4 summarizes these syndromes.

Ulnar impaction syndrome (ulnar-lunate abutment or impaction syndrome) is the most common of these disorders.[43] This condition is associated with ulnar positive variance (ulna longer than radius at the radial articular margin). Patients present with chronic wrist pain, made worse by activity and relieved by rest.[15,43] Routine radiographs demonstrate ulnar positive variance with sclerosis or cystic changes in the lunate and triquetrum. Degenerative

TABLE 4-4. ULNAR-SIDED IMPACTION SYNDROMES[15,43]

Ulnar impaction syndrome: chronic impaction of ulnar head, TFC, and adjacent lunate and triquetrum
Ulnar carpal impaction syndrome due to ulnar styloid nonunion: un-united fragment acts as loose body
Ulnar styloid impaction syndrome: chronic impaction of abnormally long ulnar styloid on the triquetrum
Ulnar impingement (impaction) syndrome: shortened ulna impinges on the distal radius
Hamatolunate impaction syndrome: due to type II lunate leading to arthrosis and chronic impingement with the wrist in ulnar deviation

TFC, triangular fibrocartilage.

TFC tears (Palmer type II) are common.[63] Coronal MR images more clearly demonstrate the TFC and osseous changes (Fig. 4-18).[43] Focal signal abnormality is evident in the lunate in 87%, the radial aspect of the triquetrum in 43%, and the radial aspect of the ulnar head in 10% of patients.[43] Though the ulnar length is usually increased on MR images, the measurement should be made on neutral posteroanterior wrist radiographs. It is difficult to obtain the appropriate position when performing MR examinations.[15]

Ulnocarpal impaction syndrome (Table 4-4) is due to an un-united ulnar styloid fracture. The fragment may act as a loose body causing adjacent carpal irritation and arthrosis or impingement on the ECU tendon. There may also be associated tears of the TFC.[15,43]

Routine radiographs will demonstrate the fracture in most cases. Care must be taken not to confuse accessory ossicles for an un-united fracture. When there is ECU involvement, focal swelling along the ulnar styloid may be evident. MRI is an excellent technique for evaluating the osseous changes and ECU involvement (Figs. 4-19 and 4-20).[10,11,15]

Ulnar styloid impaction syndrome is due to an elongated ulnar styloid that causes chronic triquetral impaction.

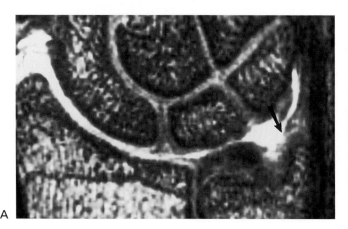
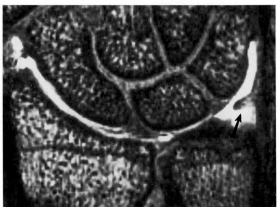

FIGURE 4-17. Coronal gradient echo arthrogram images **(A, B)** demonstrating a triangular fibrocartilage tear near the ulnar attachment *(arrow)*.

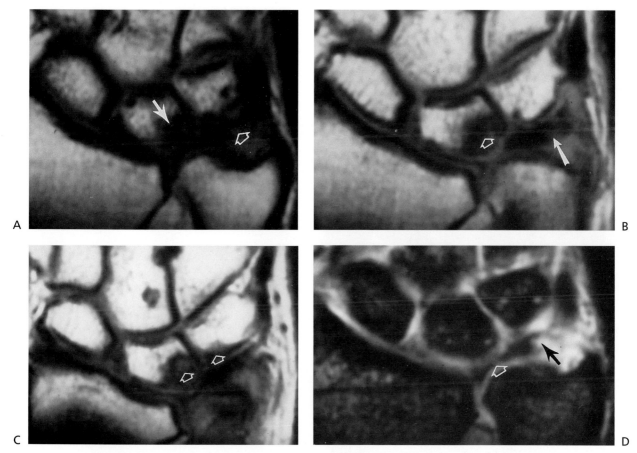

FIGURE 4-18. Ulnar impaction (ulnar-lunate impaction) syndrome. **A:** Coronal T1-weighted image with a large lunate defect *(arrow),* ulnar positive variance, and a triangular fibrocartilage (TFC) tear *(open arrow).* **B, C:** Coronal T1-weighted images demonstrate ulnar elongation, a TFC tear *(arrow)* and signal abnormality in the lunate and triquetrum *(open arrows).* **D:** Coronal T2-weighted sequence demonstrates ulnar positive variance with elevation of the radial aspect of the TFC *(open arrow)* and a peripheral tear *(arrow).*

This disorder is usually definable on radiographs (Fig. 4-12). However, secondary changes are more easily appreciated using MRI.[15]

Two additional causes of ulnar-sided wrist pain include ulnar impingement and hamate-lunate impaction syndrome. The former is due to impingement of a shortened ulna on the radius.[15] Hamate-lunate impaction is associated with a type II lunate, which may be evident in up to 50% of patients. Up to 25% of patients with a medial facet that articulates with the hamate develop chondromalacia and arthrosis.[15] These changes are more easily appreciated on coronal T1- and T2-weighted images.[11]

Treatment of these disorders may involve arthroscopic or open procedures. Ulnar shortening (Fig. 4-21) may be required in patients with ulnar positive variance.[15,43]

Ligament Injury/Instability

Carpal instability can be seen following ligament tears, following fracture with improper healing, and in association with inflammatory arthropathies.[10,33,70] Ligament tears may involve the intrinsic interosseous ligaments or extrinsic dorsal and palmar ligament complexes as well as the radioulnar complex. The metacarpophalangeal (MCP) and phalangeal ligaments may also be disrupted.[10,67,68]

Disruption of the radioulnar ligaments (Fig. 4-22) and TFC complex can result in ulnar translation of the carpus and subluxation or dislocation of the DRUJ depending on the structures involved.[10,62,63]

Several carpal collapse patterns have been described. These patterns can be easily defined on radiographs (posteroanterior and lateral).[10] Dorsal intercalated segment instability (DISI) is most common and results in an increased scapholunate angle (normal 45°) on lateral radiographs (Fig. 4-23) with the scaphoid in a more palmar flexed position and the lunate tilted dorsally. The capitate also shifts dorsally. The DISI pattern is associated with scapholunate ligament and volar extrinsic ligament disruptions.[10,33] Volar intercalated segment instability (VISI) is seen less frequently. With this pattern, the scapholunate angle is reduced. The

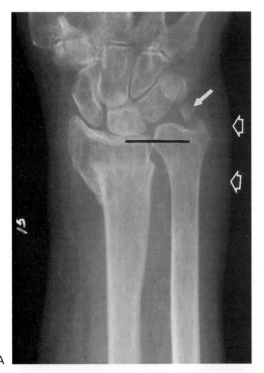

A

FIGURE 4-19. (A) Posteroanterior radiograph demonstrates an old distal radial fracture with shortening. There is significant ulnar positive variance and an un-united ulnar styloid *(arrow)*. There is also swelling *(open arrows)* along the course of the extensor carpi ulnaris (ECU) tendon. Axial T1-weighted **(B)** and proton density **(C)** images demonstrate marked thickening of the ECU with tenosynovitis *(arrow)*.

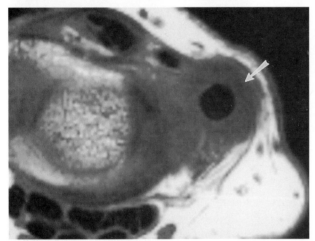

B

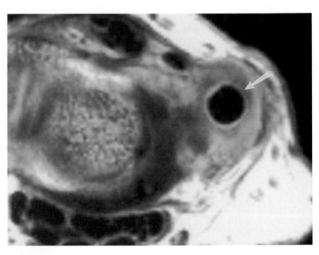

C

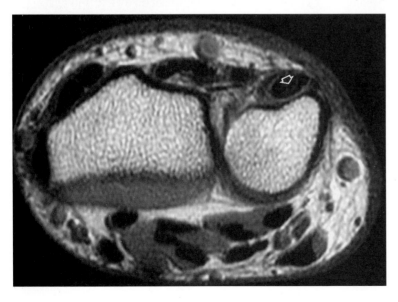

FIGURE 4-20. Axial 3T T1-weighted image shows slight subluxation, thickening and subtle signal abnormality *(open arrow)* due to extensor carpi ulnaris tendonosis.

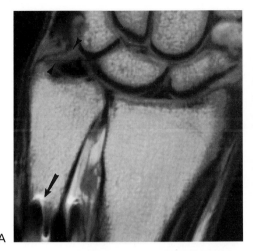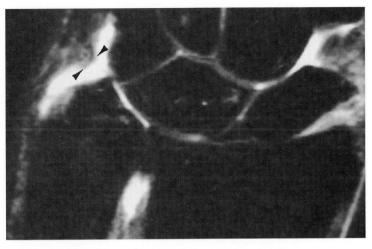

FIGURE 4-21. Ulnar shortening. Coronal T1-weighted **(A)** and fat-suppressed T2-weighted fast spin echo **(B)** images show artifact *(arrow)* from the ulnar shortening and a persistent triangular fibrocartilage tear *(arrowheads)*.

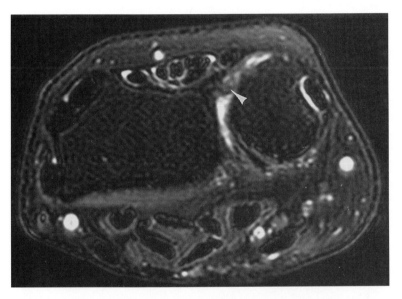

FIGURE 4-22. Axial 3T fast spin-echo with fat suppression demonstrates a surgically confirmed tear *(arrowhead)* of the dorsal distal radioulnar ligament.

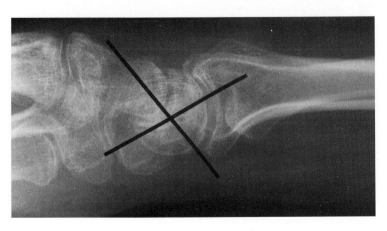

FIGURE 4-23. Dorsal intercalated segment instability pattern on the lateral radiograph with increased scapholunate angle, the lunate tilted dorsally and the capitate shifted dorsally.

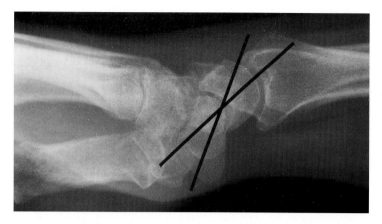

FIGURE 4-24. Ventral intercalated segment instability pattern on the lateral radiograph with the lunate tilted volarly and a decreased scapholunate angle.

lunate is in palmar flexion and palmar shift of the capitate (Fig. 4-24). The VISI pattern is seen with lunotriquetral and dorsal extrinsic ligament tears and in association with rheumatoid arthritis.[4,10,33] Scapholunate advanced collapse (SLAC) is seen with posttraumatic arthropathy. Scapholunate ligament tears as well as radioscaphoid and scaphotrazeotrapezoid degenerative disease are common.[33] These patterns can be identified on MR images (sagittal and coronal), but identification is more difficult and wrist positioning is critical.[11,76,92] Scapholunate angles tend to be increased in comparison with standard radiographs, which could lead to false-positive studies.[92] These changes are especially common when the wrist is in slight ulnar or radial deviation (Fig. 4-25).[4,92]

Ligament injuries to the MCP joints, especially the thumb, also occur.[3,51,68] Interphalangeal ligament injuries without associated dislocation are uncommon.[10]

Imaging of ligament injuries to the hand and wrist should begin with routine radiography.[10] Subtle or obvious changes in position, collapse patterns, bony erosions, and soft-tissue changes may suggest or in some cases make the diagnosis.[10,11] Prior to MRI, arthrography with or without stress views was used to diagnose or confirm suspected ligament injuries to the hand and wrist.[10,68] Today MRI or MRA is most commonly employed in this setting. The imaging technique selected depends on the clinical indications and need for diagnostic or therapeutic injections in addition to imaging studies. The latter are useful to confirm the source of pain.[10]

Distal Radioulnar Joint

DRUJ instability is a common cause of wrist pain following trauma, radial shortening after fracture, and inflammatory

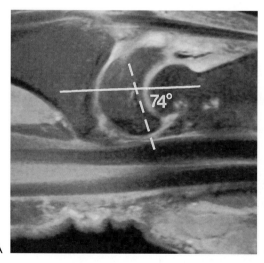

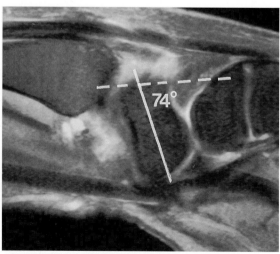

FIGURE 4-25. Sagittal fat-suppressed postcontrast T1-weighted images **(A, B)** of the wrist with the patient in slight ulnar deviation. Measurement of the scapholunate angle on these two images *(lines and dotted lines)* results in an increased angle of 74° (normal 45°). Note the lunate is not tilted dorsally.

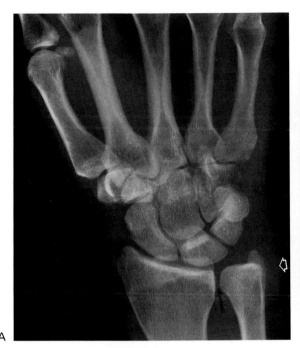
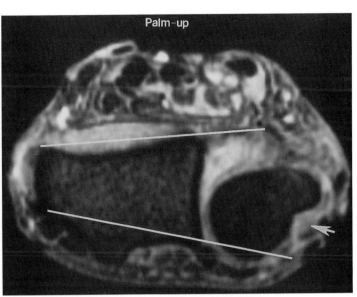

FIGURE 4-26. Subluxation of the distal radioulnar joint (DRUJ). **A:** Posteroanterior radiograph shows swelling along the ulna *(open arrow)* and slight widening of the DRUJ *(arrow)*. **B:** Axial gradient echo with the palm up shows subluxation *(lines)* of the DRUJ and an absent extensor carpi ulnaris due to complete disruption *(arrow)*.

arthropathies such as rheumatoid arthritis.[10,84] In routine radiography this injury is frequently overlooked unless significant subluxation or joint widening is evident.[10] Either CT or MRI can be performed to confirm DRUJ subluxation. However, technique is important to ensure optimal accuracy.[10,57,84] Axial images can be obtained with the patient in neutral, supine, or prone position through the DRUJ.[57] Cine-looped motion studies are also possible.[84] Contrast injection of the DRUJ may be useful to access the ligaments (see Fig. 4-22) and TFC complex, but contrast is not essential to confirm subluxation.[11] Noncontrast MR images can be obtained using T1-weighted and T2-weighted (spin echo or FSE with fat suppression) or T2* gradient echo images (Fig. 4-26).[10,11,84] All positions should be evaluated. Keep in mind that the ulna may look slightly dorsally subluxed when the hand is palm down.[4,11]

Scapholunate Ligament

The normal appearance of the scapholunate ligament varies with the portion included in the image plane. The ligament is "C" shaped extending from the dorsal to proximal to volar aspects of the scapholunate articulation (Fig. 4-27). Thus, the distal joint space allows contrast to extend between the scaphoid and lunate to the level of the proximal ligament. No contrast should extend into the radiocarpal joint.[10,11] On coronal images the appearance varies in the volar, middle, and dorsal portions of the ligament. The volar portion usually is trapezoidal in configuration. The central portion (proximal) is triangular and may have inhomogeneous signal intensity. The dorsal portion is typically band-like in appearance (Fig. 4-27B).[70,74,88]

Conventional and MR arthropathic approaches have been used to evaluate the scapholunate ligament.[4,11,76,85] Conventional spin echo or FSE sequences can identify the ligament. Appearance obviously varies with different pulse sequences. In most cases the ligament is low signal intensity. Most studies and the best conventional imaging approach uses 1-mm-thick three-dimensional gradient echo sequences.[11,74,78,88] Totterman and Miller[88] described the scapholunate ligament appearance (Fig. 4-27B) in the volar, middle, and dorsal planes on coronal three-dimensional gradient echo images (69/15, FA 20°, 256 × 256 matrix, one acquisition, 8-cm FOV). The volar portion of the ligament is trapezoidal with inhomogeneous signal intensity on MR images. The inhomogeneity had a striated appearance.[88] The midportion (proximal) of the scapholunate ligament is triangular with inhomogeneous low to intermediate signal intensity. The dorsal portion of the ligament is band-like with low to intermediate inhomogeneous signal intensity.[88] When the ligament attaches to cartilage, the signal intensity is increased at the margin which should not be confused with a tear. Signal intensity at bone attachments is low.[78] The higher signal intensity of the volar portion of the ligament may be due to loose collagen fibers and vascular tissue compared with the more dense collagen in the middle and dorsal portions.[78,88]

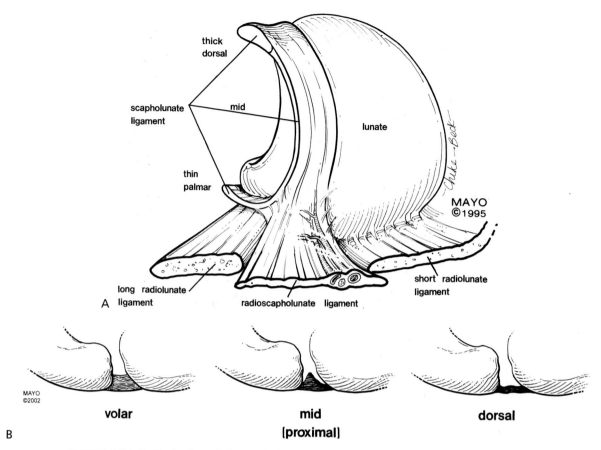

FIGURE 4-27. A: Illustration of the scapholunate ligament seen from the radial side with the scaphoid removed. (From Berger RA. Ligament anatomy. In: Cooney WP, Linscheid RL, Dobyns JH, eds. The wrist: diagnosis and operative treatment. St. Louis: Mosby, 1998:32–60.) **B:** Illustration of the configuration changes in the scapholunate ligament seen on coronal MR images in the dorsal, middle, and volar portions.

Smith[78] found the scapholunate ligament to be low intensity in 63% but with areas of intermediate signal intensity in 37% of those examined. He described the ligament as linear or triangular depending on the level of section. Signal intensity was low and uniform in 49% (type I). Type II increased signal (Fig. 4-28) occurred in 14%, type III increased signal (Fig. 4-28) occurred distally and type IV proximally. Intermediate signal extended through the ligament in 19% (type V) (Fig. 4-28).[78]

Scapholunate ligament tears may be seen as a linear area of increased signal intensity.[11,70] Fragmentation, absence of the ligament, and widening of the scapholunate space may also be evident (Fig. 4-29).[11,70,74,75] The extent of the tear is important to evaluate on all images. Though controversial, Berger[9] showed that when the middle (proximal) portion was involved, instability was not always present. Tears that include the dorsal portion result in instability.[9] Accuracy of conventional MRI for detection of scapholunate tears has varied from 77% to 87%.[11,70,74] Sensitivities and specificities range from 50% to 93% and from 86% to 100%, respectively.[70]

Magnetic resonance arthrography is more accurate (see Figs. 4-28B, C and 4-30). Radiocarpal injections are usually adequate (Fig. 4-28B, C). On occasion, midcarpal injections add information regarding partial distal surface tears. Fat-suppressed T1-weighted and three-dimensional gradient echo sequences are obtained after intra-articular injection.[11] This permits evaluation of all three portions of the ligament in 95% of cases.[59] Scheck et al.[74] reported accurate detection of tears in 94% of patients on MR arthrograms. Sensitivities and specificities were 52% and 34% for conventional MRI compared with 90% and 87% for MRA.

Lunotriquetral Ligament

The lunotriquetral ligament, like the scapholunate ligament, is "C" shaped.[10,11] The ligament spans the dorsal, proximal and volar aspects of the lunotriquetral articulation. Therefore, contrast from the midcarpal joint can extend to the proximal aspect of the ligament but should not enter the radiocarpal joint. Similar to the scapholunate ligament, a membranous and fibrocartilaginous triangular portion

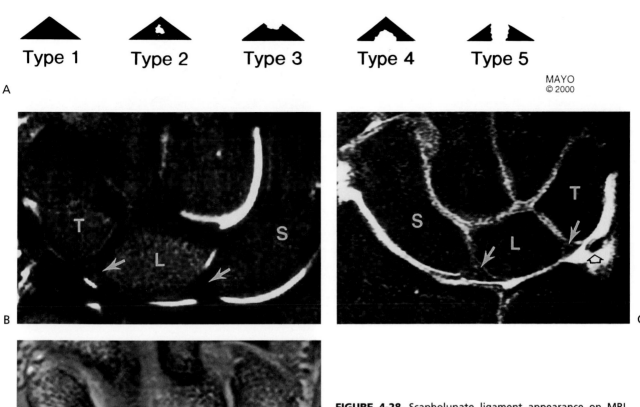

A

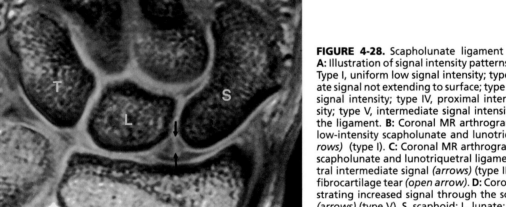

B

C

D

FIGURE 4-28. Scapholunate ligament appearance on MRI. A: Illustration of signal intensity patterns described by Smith.[78] Type I, uniform low signal intensity; type II, central intermediate signal not extending to surface; type III, distal intermediate signal intensity; type IV, proximal intermediate signal intensity; type V, intermediate signal intensity extending through the ligament. B: Coronal MR arthrogram showing triangular low-intensity scapholunate and lunotriquetral ligaments *(arrows)* (type I). C: Coronal MR arthrogram showing triangular scapholunate and lunotriquetral ligaments with areas of central intermediate signal *(arrows)* (type II). Note the triangular fibrocartilage tear *(open arrow)*. D: Coronal MR image demonstrating increased signal through the scapholunate ligament *(arrows)* (type V). S, scaphoid; L, lunate; T, triquetrum.

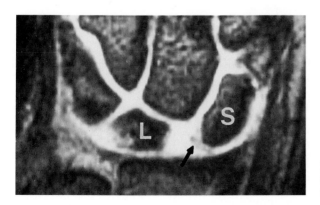

FIGURE 4-29. Conventional T2-weighted coronal MR image shows widening of the scapholunate space with a ligament fragment *(arrow)* near the scaphoid attachment. S, scaphoid; L, lunate.

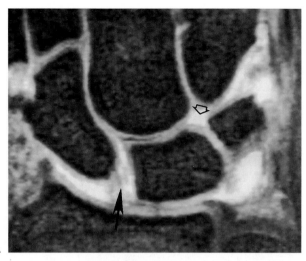
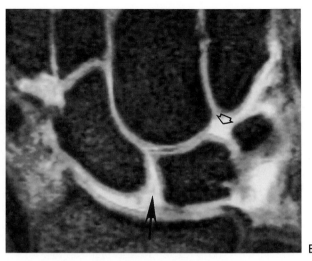

FIGURE 4-30. Coronal postradiocarpal arthrogram images **(A, B)** demonstrate subtle widening of the scapholunate joint compared to the lunotriquetral. There is contrast in the intercarpal joint *(open arrow)* with increased signal in the scapholunate ligament *(arrow)*. Differentiating scapholunate from lunotriquetral tears in this setting could be difficult if the injection were not monitored fluoroscopically.

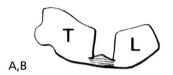

FIGURE 4-31. Configuration of the lunotriquetral ligament on MR images. **A:** Triangular 63%; **B:** linear 37%; **C:** amorous. L, lunate; T, triquetrum.

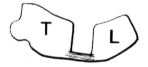
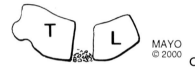
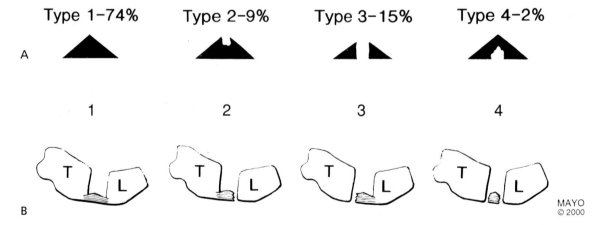

FIGURE 4-32. Signal intensity variations described by Smith.[79] **A:** Type I, homogeneous low intensity 74%; type II, distal intermediate signal intensity 9%; type III, linear increased intensity signal through the ligament 15%; type IV, proximal linear increased signal intensity 2%. **B:** Signal intensity may also vary at the bony attachments. (1) normal, (2) cleft at lunate attachment, (3) cleft at triquetral attachment, (4) clefts at both attachments. L, lunate; T, triquetrum.

extends between the articular surfaces.[79,88] The appearance of the lunotriquetral ligament also varies in different coronal planes with variations in signal intensity and shape similar to those described with the scapholunate ligament (Fig. 4-28B, C).[70,79]

Smith[79] also described variations in the lunotriquetral ligament. The lunotriquetral ligament is triangular in 63% and linear in 37% of patients. This obviously varies with the plane of section (Fig. 4-31).[11,78] Signal intensity varies (Fig. 4-32) similar to the scapholunate ligament. Signal intensity changes are also described at the bony attachments.[79]

Detection of lunotriquetral ligament tears can be accomplished with radiocarpal or midcarpal arthrography (Fig. 4-13).[11] There is a high incidence of lunotriquetral tears associated with TFC complex tears (70%). Therefore when the DRUJ is injected, both tears may be evident on one injection (Fig. 4-13).[10] Routine radiographs may show articular step-off or overlap, but the space is not increased as seen with scapholunate ligament tears. Keep in mind that asymptomatic perforations may be noted in 13% of patients older than 40 years.[10,79]

Lunotriquetral ligament tears may be partial or complete (Fig. 4-33). Partial tears may require two-compartment (radiocarpal and midcarpal) injections for evaluation whether conventional or MR arthrography is used.[10]

Conventional MRI is less accurate for evaluating the lunotriquetral ligament than the scapholunate ligament. Sensitivity and specificity range from 40% to 56% and from 45% to 100%, respectively.[70] The use of MRA improves accuracy.

Extrinsic Ligaments

Evaluation of the dorsal and volar ligaments of the wrist is more complex. Tears of these ligaments are often associated

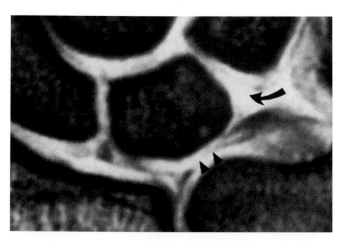

FIGURE 4-33. Coronal gradient echo image demonstrating a lunotriquetral tear (curved arrow) and a triangular fibrocartilage tear *(double arrowheads)* with ulnar positive variance and lunate chondromalacia. (From Oneson SR, Timins ME, Scales LM, et al. MR diagnosis of triangular fibrocartilage pathology with arthroscopic correlation. AJR 1997;168:1513–1518.)

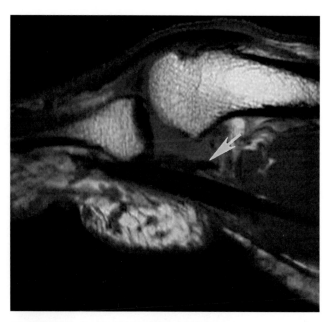

FIGURE 4-34. Sagittal T1-weighted 3T image demonstrates volar subluxation of the metacarpophalangeal joint with avulsion *(arrow)* of the volar plate.

with other osseous and soft-tissue injuries.[10] Multiple image planes or three-dimensional reconstructions can identify the volar and dorsal ligaments.[2,80,81] To date, there are no reliable data on the accuracy of MRI or MRA for detection of tears in these structures.

Metacarpophalangeal/Interphalangeal Ligaments

Injuries may also occur involving the ligament support of the MCP and phalangeal joints.[10,38,67] Injuries may be associated with fracture or dislocation, or they may occur as isolated events (Fig. 4-34). We will focus on injury to the ulnar collateral ligament (UCL) of the first MCP joint as it occurs commonly. The injury was originally termed "gamekeeper's thumb" because it occurred in Scottish gamekeepers as a result of the method used to kill rabbits.[3] Nowadays the injury is common in skiers where it accounts for 6% to 9.5% of all skiing injuries.[38,51,68,89]

The fibrocartilaginous palmar plate is thin proximally and thick distally. The sesamoids are located in the volar plate at the insertions of the flexor pollicis brevis and adductor brevis.[10,68] The UCL arises from the medial tubercle of the metacarpal condyle and takes an oblique anterior course to insert on the base of the proximal phalanx near the volar plate.[3,68] The UCL is the major stabilizer of the ulnar side of the thumb. The adductor pollicis has three insertions, including the ulnar sesamoid and palmar plate, the lateral tubercle of the proximal phalanx, and the dorsal expansion.[68] The insertion confluent with the dorsal expansion hood and superficial to the UCL is termed the adductor aponeurosis.[10,68]

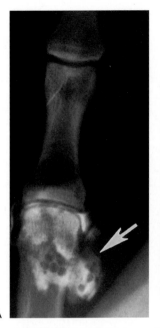
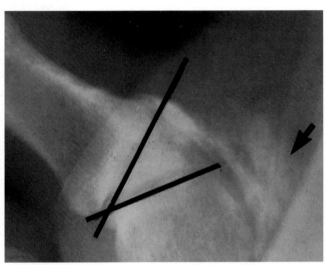

A   B

FIGURE 4-35. Arthrograms of the first metacarpophalangeal joint. **A:** Posteroanterior unstressed image demonstrates extravasation *(arrow)* due to an ulnar collateral ligament and capsule tear. **B:** Stress radiograph shows contrast extravasation due to the ligament tear and opening of the joint on the ulnar side.

Injury to the UCL occurs with forced abduction of the thumb. Tears most commonly occur near the distal phalangeal insertion.[3,38,51] When displaced the ligament can retract and displace so that it lies superficial to the adductor aponeurosis. This is called the Stener lesion.[3,51,89] Identification of Stener lesions is important because they require surgical repair.[3] Failure to diagnose UCL lesions results in instability and early arthrosis.[3,68]

Diagnosis of ulnar collateral ligament tears may be suspected clinically and confirmed with stress arthrography (Fig. 4-35).[10,38,68] Anesthetic injection is important in the acute setting due to pain, which could prevent adequate application of stress. Both thumbs are usually stressed for comparison.[10] MRI and MRA have replaced arthrography at many institutions in recent years.[3,38,40,51,89] Arthrography demonstrated 83% of tears but only 61% of displaced tears. Conventional MRI demonstrated 90% and MRA 100% of displaced tears (Fig. 4-36).[3]

TENDON INJURIES

A review of tendon anatomy is important in order to properly plan and interpret imaging studies of the hand and wrist.[11,17] A knowledge of surgical landmarks is also important.[10]

The flexor tendons begin in the distal third of the forearm.[10] At the wrist, the flexor pollicis longus passes the flexor retinaculum and is enclosed in its own tendon sheath (radial bursa). The flexor digitorum profundus and super-

ficialis tendons lie dorsal and medial to the median nerve and are enclosed in a common tendon sheath (ulnar bursa) (Fig. 4-37).[10] The relationships of the flexor tendons to the MCP and proximal interphalangeal (PIP) joints is also important.[17] At the MCP joint the flexor tendon lies just palmar to the volar plate in the A1 pulley (Fig. 4-38). It has a similar position at the PIP joint in the A3 pulley.[10,17,24,32] Zones have been described for surgical planning following flexor tendon injuries. It is important for imagers to be aware of these zones (Fig. 4-37) and to correlate them with the site of injury.[11]

The extensor tendons are stabilized by six dorsal compartments at the wrist (Fig. 4-39).[10,11,17] At the level of the extensor retinaculum, the tendons are enclosed in tendon sheaths (Fig. 4-34).[10,17,23] Just proximal to the MCP joints the extensor digitorum communis tendons are joined together by the junctura tendinum.[10,17,23]

The relationship of the extensor tendons to the MCP, PIP, and DIP joints are summarized in Figs. 4-38A, B and 4-39B. As with the flexor tendons, zones are established for the extensor tendons for surgical planning purposes (Fig. 4-40).[11,17,23]

Injuries to the tendons of the hand and wrist occur commonly (Table 4-5).[8,10-12,28,33,70] Inflammation of the tendon (tendonitis) or tendon sheath (tenosynovitis) or perivascular bundle (peritendonitis) may occur alone or in combination. Tendonosis is a degenerative process seen with overuse and age that results in mucoid degeneration, vascular ingrowth, and cartilage metaplasia.[70] Rupture of the tendons may be partial or complete.[11,64,73]

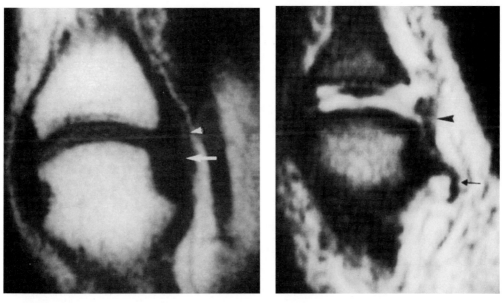

FIGURE 4-36. MRI in gamekeeper's thumb. **A:** Coronal SE 600/20 image demonstrating a normal ulnar collateral ligament *(arrow)* and adductor pollicis aponeurosis *(arrowhead)*. **B:** Coronal SE 2000/80 image demonstrating a Stener lesion with proximally retracted torn ulnar collateral ligament *(arrow)* with respect to the adductor pollicis aponeurosis *(arrowhead)*. (From Harper MT, Chandnani VP, Spaeth J, et al. Gamekeeper thumb: diagnosis of ulnar collateral ligament injury using magnetic resonance imaging, magnetic resonance arthrography, and stress radiography. J Magn Reson Imaging 1996;6:322–328.)

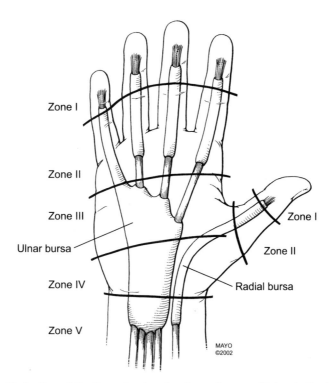

FIGURE 4-37. Illustration of the flexor tendon sheaths and zones of injury in the hand and wrist.

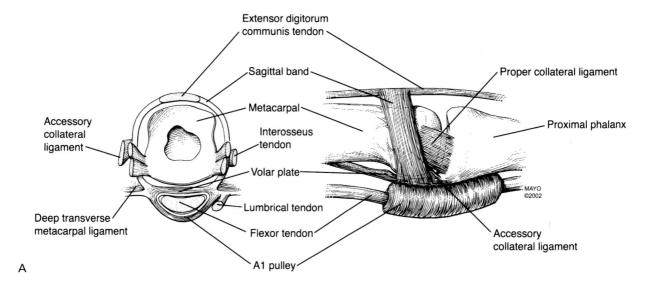

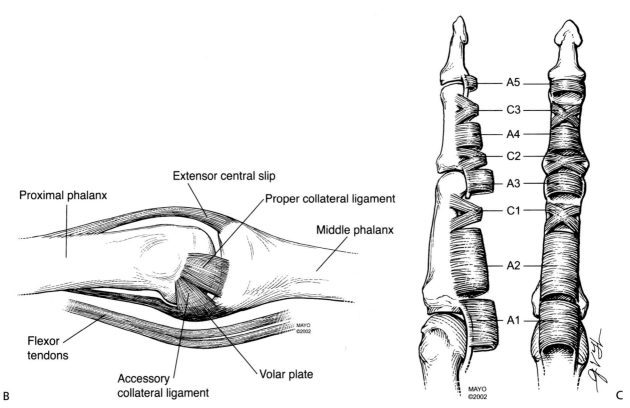

FIGURE 4-38. **A:** Illustration of the flexor and extensor tendons seen in the axial and lateral planes in relation to the metacarpophalangeal joint. **B:** Illustration of the flexor and extensor tendons at the proximal interphalangeal joint. **C:** Illustration of the pulley system for the flexor tendons. There are five annular **(A)** and three "C"-shaped **(C)** pulleys that allow the sheath to conform to position with flexion.

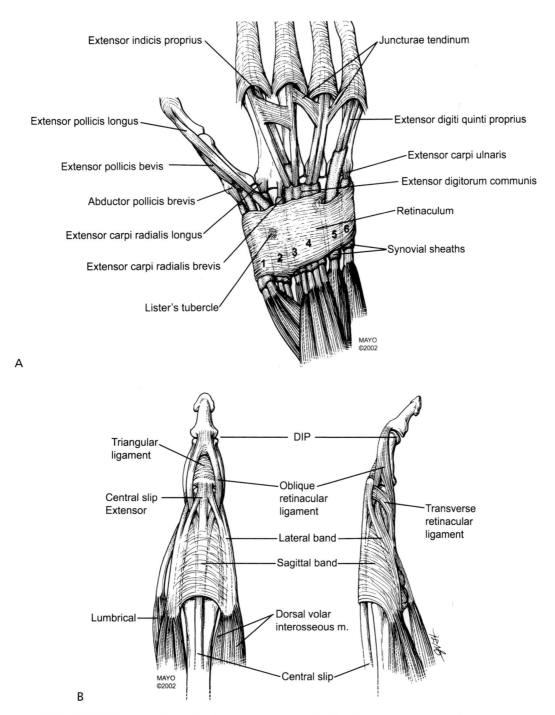

FIGURE 4-39. A: Illustration of extensor tendons, tendon sheaths, and the six dorsal compartments. **B:** Illustration of the extensor tendons in the finger seen dorsally and laterally.

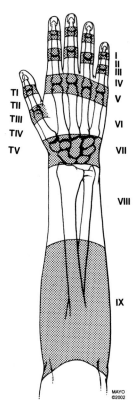

FIGURE 4-40. Illustration of zones for extensor tendon surgical repair.

Patients with tendon injuries present with pain and diminished function involving the affected tendon or tendons. Prior to MRI, clinical diagnosis or tenography was used to evaluate tendon disorders of the hand and wrist.[10,39,70] Routine radiography is still an important screening examination to exclude bone avulsion or other subtle changes that may suggest the diagnosis.[10,16,39]

Conventional MRI and MR tenography are frequently used today for the diagnosis and grading of tendon injuries.[10–12,28,33] Normal tendons are low signal intensity

TABLE 4-5. TENDON DISORDERS: MRI FEATURES

Condition	MR Features
Tendinosis	Intermediate ↑ signal intensity proton density and T2-weighted sequences, tendon thickening
Tendinitis	Intermediate signal intensity proton density with high signal on T2-weighted sequence, tendon thickening
Tenosynovitis	↑ signal intensity surrounding tendon on T2-weighted sequences. Tendon signal intensity normal
Partial tear	↑ signal intensity and thickening T2-weighted sequences
Complete tear	↑ signal intensity with tendon segments separated. Retracted tendon may be serpiginous

on all MR sequences.[10,11,33] There is normally minimal fluid in the tendon sheath. When fluid completely surrounds the tendon, inflammation is likely. Inflammatory changes in the tendon sheath and tendon are most easily demonstrated on T2-weighted sequences (Table 4-5; Fig. 4-41).[4,10,11,33] Tendon inflammation and partial tears show increased signal intensity and thickening in the area of involvement (Fig. 4-42). Signal intensity increases on T2-weighted sequences compared with proton density (intermediate signal intensity) with inflammation and partial tears. In general, with tendonosis signal intensity does not increase significantly on T2-weighted sequences (Table 4-5).[11,70] The tendon ends are separated and may be retracted with complete tears. Increased signal intensity is noted between the segments, and tendons may have a serpiginous appearance with complete tears on T2-weighted sequences (Table 4-5; Fig. 4-43).[11,49]

As experience with the use of MRI in hand and wrist disorders has increased, more data have become available regarding the application of MRI in the evaluation of tendonopathies. Therefore, we will focus on specific disorders where MRI provides the clinician with valuable information about diagnosis and treatment planning.

Tendon/Pulley System Ruptures

Tendon ruptures may occur with acute trauma or with overuse and degeneration. Ruptures may be partial or complete (Table 4-4).[11,70,71,83] Ruptures may also result from fracture malunion or nonunion, as well as from inflammatory arthropathies. Patients with rheumatoid arthritis develop tenosynovitis in 64% of cases. Persistent inflammation frequently leads to partial or complete disruption.[83] Rupture of the flexor pollicis longus has been described with scaphoid nonunion and rheumatoid arthritis.[73] Tendon tears in the fingers and hand occur more often with skin wounds or lacerations.[24,39]

The pulley system (Fig. 4-38C) is critical for flexor tendon function. These structures keep the flexor tendon in position along the phalanges during finger flexion.[46,64] Rupture of the pulley system may occur with forced extension when the finger is flexed. The tendon remains intact.[32,51] Pulley system rupture is associated with activities such as rock climbing.[32,46] Injury to the pulley system (Fig. 4-38C) may result in "bowstring" deformity of the flexor tendons.[31,50,63]

Zones have been developed for flexor and extensor tendon injury that provide treatment approaches (Figs. 4-37 and 4-40).[24,53,71] These regions should be kept in mind when planning imaging studies and describing the findings. Imaging should begin with routine radiographs to evaluate any osseous changes (fracture, malunion, nonunion, arthropathy, soft-tissue abnormalities).[10,11] Tendon injuries can be more completely evaluated with dynamic sonography or MRI.[11,46,83] In our practice, tendon injuries are most commonly evaluated with MRI or, rarely,

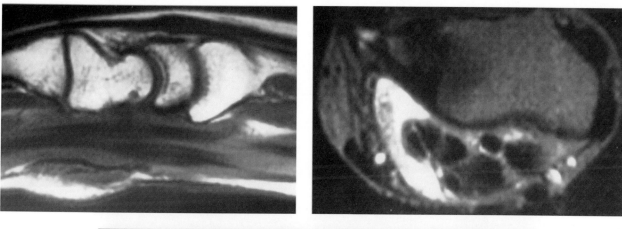

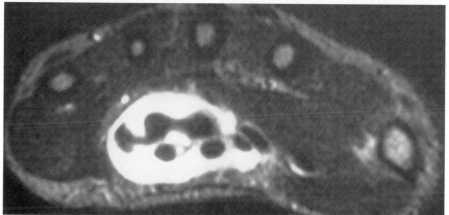

FIGURE 4-41. Sagittal T1- **(A)** and axial T2-weighted **(B, C)** spin echo sequences demonstrate flexor tenosynovitis with high intensity fluid in the tendon sheaths and normal low signal intensity tendons in a gymnast with overuse syndrome.

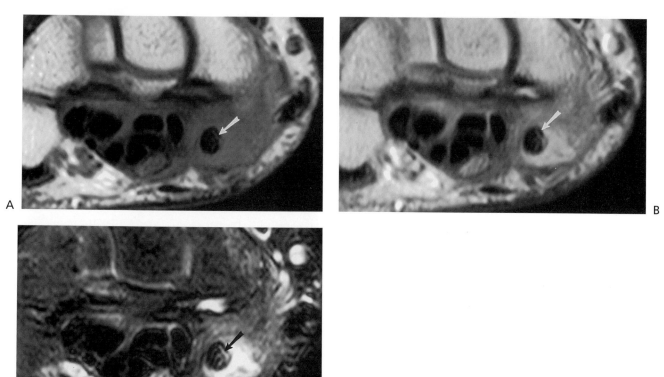

FIGURE 4-42. Axial T1-weighted **(A)**, proton density **(B)**, and T2-weighted **(C)** sequences demonstrate thickening, increased signal intensity that increased from the proton density **(B)** to T2-weighted **(C)** images *(arrow)* and surrounding fluid due to a partial tear in the flexor carpi radialis tendon.

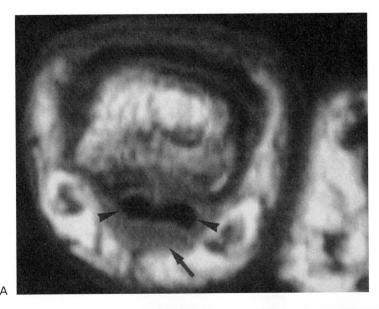

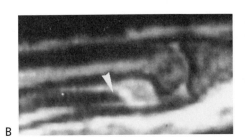

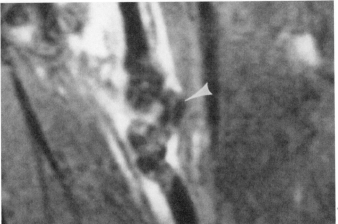

FIGURE 4-43. Flexor digitorum profundus tendon tear. **A:** Axial T1-weighted image at the proximal interphalangeal joint level shows an absent tendon in the digital canal *(arrow)*. The two segments of the flexor digitorum superficialis are evident *(arrowheads)*. **B:** Gradient echo image shows the tendon tear and retraction at the C2 pulley level *(arrowhead)*. **C:** Coronal image shows the curled tendon in the palm *(arrowhead)*. (From Drapé J-L, deGery S T-C, Silbermann-Hoffman O, et al. Closed ruptures of the flexor digitorum tendons: MRI evaluation. Skel Radiol 1998;27: 617–624.)

MR tenography.[10,11,24,39,71] Image planes used most commonly are axial and sagittal for the fingers, axial and coronal for the hand, and axial and coronal or sagittal for the wrist. Sagittal images in flexion and extension are indicated when pulley system injuries are suspected (Fig. 4-44).[11,64] T2-weighted sequences (spin echo, or fat-suppressed fast spin echo) with 3-mm sections, 8-cm FOV, 1 acquisition, and 256 × 256 matrix are used. Volume gradient echo three-dimensional images can be obtained in the coronal plane for wrist evaluation. Tenography is useful to more clearly define the pulley systems.[39]

Flexor tendon disruptions occur most commonly. Convention studies are usually adequate in the hand and wrist. Tenography may be important for complete evaluation of the tendons in the fingers and injury to the pulley system (Fig. 4-44).[39] Kumar et al.[49] graded flexor tendon injury. Type I injuries show retraction of the proximal segment into the hand, resulting in loss of vascular supply to the tendon ends (Fig. 4-43C). Type II ruptures have the proximal end retracted to the PIP joint level. Vascular supply is preserved in this setting. Type III injuries are associated with an avulsed bone fragment.[49] Surgical reattachment is not successful if type I lesions are not diagnosed acutely. Type II lesions may be successfully repaired after delay in diagnosis of several months due to intact blood supply (Figs. 4-45 and 4-46).[49]

Ruptures of the pulley system can be diagnosed by "bowstringing" with the finger flexed (Fig. 4-47).[32,39,64,83] Tenography optimizes evaluation.[39]

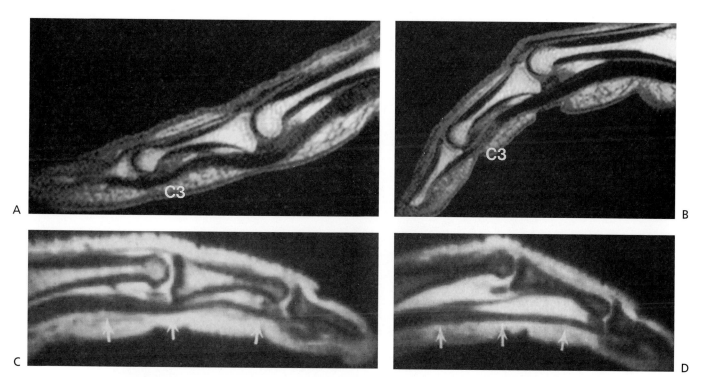

A   B

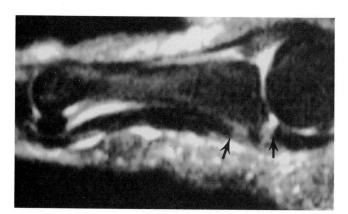

C   D

FIGURE 4-44. Pulley system rupture. Sagittal T1-weighted images in the extended **(A)** and flexed **(B)** positions demonstrating an intact pulley system with normal relationship of the flexor tendon to the phalanges maintained. Note signal intensity change at the C3 level with flexion. Question magic angle or partial volume effect. T1-weighted extended **(C)** and flexed **(D)** in a patient with pulley system rupture. The flexor tendon is mildly separated from the phalanx in extension *(arrows)* **(C)**, but there is obvious bow stringing with flexion *(arrows)* **(D)**. (C and D from Bowers WH, Kuzma AR, Byrum DK. Closed traumatic rupture of finger flexor pulleys. J Hand Surg 1994;19A:782–787.)

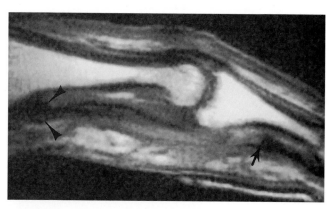

FIGURE 4-45. Sagittal fat-suppressed fast spin echo T2-weighted image of a minimally displace *(arrows)* flexor tendon rupture at the metacarpophalangeal joint level.

FIGURE 4-46. Sagittal T1-weighted image of a tendon laceration at the mid middle phalanx level *(arrow)*. The proximal tendon has retracted to the base of the proximal phalanx *(arrowheads)*. It is essential to demonstrate both tendon segments, which may require additional images or a larger field of view.

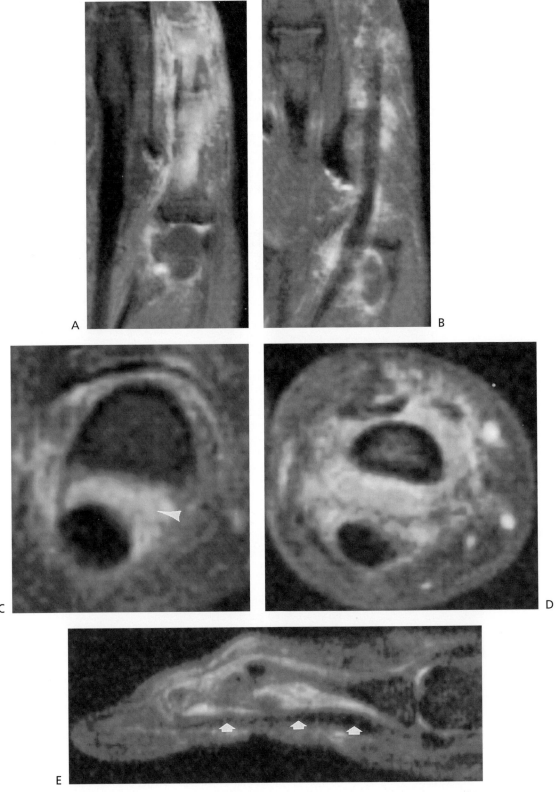

FIGURE 4-47. Pulley system rupture. Contrast-enhanced images of the fifth finger. Coronal images **(A, B)** demonstrate inflammation with enhancement along the intact flexor tendon. Axial images **(C, D)** demonstrate tendon separation from the phalanx and a defect *(arrowhead)* in the A4 pulley. Sagittal image demonstrates tendon displacement at the C1, A3, C2, A4, and C3 levels *(arrows)* **(E)**.

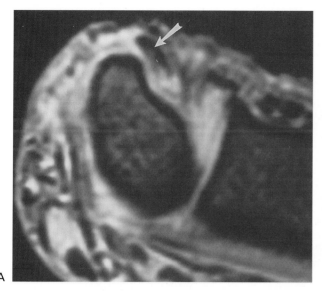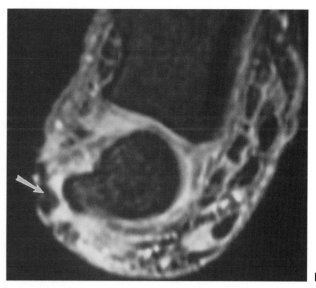

A   B

FIGURE 4-48. Axial gradient echo images at the level of the distal radioulnar joint demonstrating subluxation **(A)** progressing to dislocation **(B)** of the extensor carpi ulnaris tendon *(arrow)*.

Tendon Subluxation/Dislocation

Subluxation or dislocation of the tendons in the hand and wrist may occur with acute trauma, previous fracture with osseous deformity, inflammatory arthropathies, and overuse syndromes. Patients may have subtle symptoms or present with pain, swelling, and reduced function depending on the tendon or tendons involved.[10,11,83]

Imaging should include radiographic screening to evaluate osseous structures, joint deformity, and areas of soft-tissue swelling. Ultrasound or MRI can be employed to evaluate tendon position. Flexion, extension, pronation, supination, or other motions and positions may be required to detect subtle abnormalities, especially in the wrist (Fig. 4-48).[11]

Magnetic resonance images can be obtained using T1- and T2-weighted sequences. The axial plane is often most useful (Figs. 4-48 and 4-49).[11] Usually coronal or sagittal images are added depending on the tendon involved.

When motion is required, gradient echo sequences are used.

Management of subluxation or dislocation may be conservative if normal position can be reestablished. When conservative treatment fails, repair of supporting ligaments may be required.[10,12]

Inflammatory Disorders

Inflammatory disorders involving the tendons are common. Tendonitis or tenosynovitis of the first dorsal compartment (de Quervain's tenosynovitis) occurs most commonly.[4,16,34] The ECU tendon is the second most common location for tenosynovitis, followed by the extensor carpi radialis, flexor carpi radialis, flexor carpi ulnaris, and extensor pollicis longus (third dorsal compartment).[10,30,34,41,65]

De Quervain's stenosing tenosynovitis involves the first dorsal compartment (Fig. 4-50). Patients present with pain

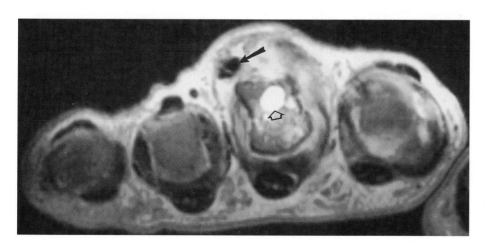

FIGURE 4-49. Inflammatory arthropathy. Axial T2-weighted image demonstrates swelling over the third metacarpophalangeal joint with dislocation of the extensor tendon *(arrow)*. There is a geode in the metacarpal head *(open arrow)*.

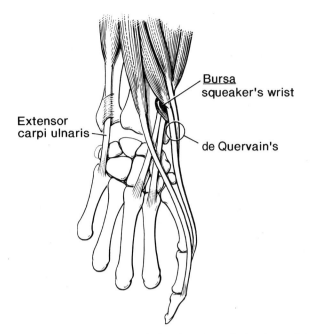

FIGURE 4-50. Illustration of the location of de Quervain's tenosynovitis and a bursa that can form just proximal to this, resulting in intersection syndrome (squeaker's wrist).

and restriction of the extensor pollicis brevis and abductor pollicis longus.[4,16] This condition is most common between the ages of 30 and 50 years.[34] Up to 77% of patients are women involved in nursing, secretarial work, or other occupations resulting in overuse (pinch, grasp, radial or ulnar deviation of the wrist) symptoms. The incidence of de Quervain's is also increased with pregnancy.[16,34] Clinically the symptoms may mimic a scaphoid fracture, flexor carpi radialis tendonitis, or degenerative arthritis at the first carpometacarpal joint, or intersection syndrome

(squeaker's wrist).[10] The last is an overuse syndrome slightly proximal to de Quervain's tendonitis (Fig. 4-50). A bursa forms between the extensor carpi radialis longus and brevis and the abductor pollicis longus and extensor pollicis brevis. Patients are usually involved in racket or rowing sports and present with pain, weak grip, and crepitation (squeaker's wrist).[10]

Routine radiographs in patients with de Quervain's tendonitis may demonstrate local soft-tissue swelling, osteopenia of the radial styloid, focal periosteal reaction, or bone erosion due to thickened inflamed synovium.[16] Multiple features have been described on MR images. Increased thickness of the extensor pollicis brevis and abductor pollicis longus tendons is the most consistent finding. Periotendinous fluid, best seen on T2-weighted sequences, is also common. Increased signal intensity in the tendons occurs less commonly.[34] A septum dividing the first dorsal compartment is present in 30% of patients with de Quervain's tendonitis.[34]

Magnetic resonance features are similar with tendonitis or tenosynovitis involving the other tendons. Inflammatory changes involving the ECU may be associated with recurrent tendon subluxation.[4] Therefore, axial images on neutral, pronation, and supination or cine motion studies should be considered to exclude subluxation (Fig. 4-48).[11]

Patients with extensor indicis proprius syndrome present with pain in the forearm and wrist with flexion of the wrist with the fingers together.[65] There is thickening on the fourth dorsal compartment and hypertrophy of the muscle.[65] Findings are easily appreciated on T1- and T2-weighted axial MR images (Fig. 4-51).

Generalized inflammatory changes in the tendons or tendon sheaths is unusual except with rheumatoid arthritis, infection, and gymnast's wrist.[31,41,83]

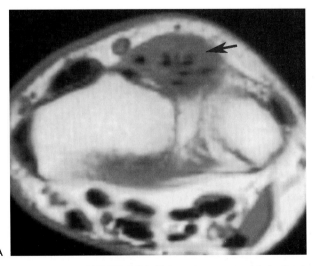
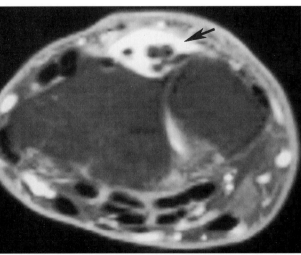

FIGURE 4-51. Extensor tenosynovitis in the fourth dorsal compartment. Axial T1-weighted **(A)** and fat-suppressed contrast-enhanced **(B)** images demonstrate tendon sheath distension in the fourth dorsal compartment *(arrow)*.

MISCELLANEOUS CONDITIONS

The previous sections have covered osseous, ligament, tendon, and TFC complex injuries. Other soft-tissue injuries may also occur, including neurovascular trauma.[11,48]

Hypothenar Hammer Syndrome

Injuries to the digital arteries are unusual.[1] However, occlusion or aneurysm formation in the distal ulnar artery near the hamate hook does occur.[48] Hypothenar hammer syndrome typically involves the dominant hand in males whose occupational activities result in chronic trauma

to this region. The syndrome has been reported in jackhammer operators, handball players, tennis players, and golfers.[11,48]

Anatomically, the ulnar artery divides into deep and superficial branches in Guyon's canal. The arteries are bounded by the pisiform and hamate hook laterally, the transverse carpal ligament dorsally, and the volar carpal ligament superficially.[50] The superficial branch of the ulnar artery penetrates the palmar aponeurosis to form the superficial palmar arch. At this point the artery is unprotected and the hamate hook serves as the anvil to which chronic trauma can compress and damage the ulnar artery proximal to the superficial palmar ulnar arch.[48,50]

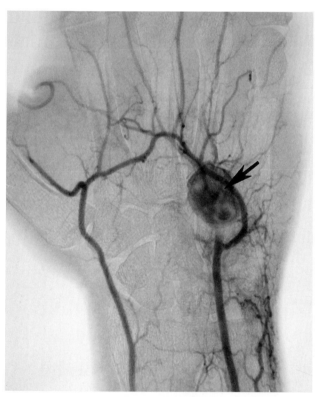

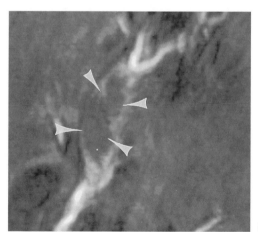

FIGURE 4-52. Posttraumatic ulnar artery aneurysms. **A:** Angiogram demonstrating a large ulnar artery aneurysm *(arrow)*. **B, C:** Axial T1-weighted MR image **(B)** demonstrates a soft-tissue mass *(arrow)* at the hamate hook. Coronal MR angiogram shows a thrombosed *(arrowheads)* ulnar artery aneurysm.

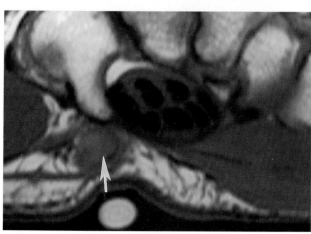

Angiography has been the gold standard for imaging the arterial system of the hand and wrist.[1,10,26] Thrombi, neural abnormalities, and aneurysms may be identified with hypothenar hammer syndrome.[48] Improvements in MR angiography have dramatically improved image quality. Therefore, MR angiography can now replace the more invasive angiographic techniques. Intravenous gadolinium is most commonly used for the hand and wrist (see Chapter 2) (Fig. 4-52).[1,11,48]

Other arterial injuries can also occur in the hand and wrist, but most are related to lacerations or open wounds.[1] An exception is frostbite injuries that result from microvascular occlusion and intracellular ice crystal formation. MRI and MR angiography can demonstrate the extent of vascular and soft-tissue disease.[6,18]

REFERENCES

1. Abouzahr MK, Coppa LM, Boxt LM. Aneurysms of the digital arteries: a case report and review of the literature. J Hand Surg 1997;22(2):311–314.
2. Adler BD, Logan PM, Janzen DL, et al. Extrinsic radiocarpal ligaments: magnetic resonance imaging of normal wrists and scapholunate dissociation. Can Assoc Radiol J 1996;47:417–422.
3. Ahn JM, Sartoris DJ, Kang HS, et al. Gamekeeper thumb: comparison of MR arthrography with conventional arthrography and MR imaging in cadavers. Radiology 1998;206:737–744.
4. Anderson MW, Kaplan PA, Dussault RG, et al. Magnetic resonance imaging of the wrist. Curr Probl Diagn Radiol 1998;Nov/Dec:191–226.
5. Arons MS, Fishbone G, Arons JA. Communicating defects in the triangular fibrocartilage complex without disruption of the triangular fibrocartilage: a report of 2 cases. J Hand Surg 1999;24A:148–151.
6. Barker JR, Haws MJ, Brown RE, et al. Magnetic resonance imaging of severe frostbite injuries. Ann Plast Surg 1997;38:275–279.
7. Beatty E, Light TR, Bedsole RJ, et al. Wrist and hand skeletal injuries in children. Hand Clin 1990;6:723–738.
8. Bengston K, Schutt AH, Swee RG, et al. Musicians overuse syndrome: a pilot study for magnetic resonance imaging. Med Prob Perf Artists 1993;8:77–80.
9. Berger RA, Imaedo T, Berglund L, et al. The anatomic constraint and material properties of the scapholunate interosseous ligament. In: Schind F, ed. Advances in biomechanics of the hand and wrist. New York: Plenum Publishing, 1994.
10. Berquist TH. Imaging of orthopedic trauma, 2nd ed. New York: Raven Press, 1992:749–870.
11. Berquist TH. MRI of the musculoskeletal system, 4th ed. Philadelphia: Lippincott Williams & Wilkins, 2001:773–841.
12. Bishop AT, Gabel G, Carmichael SW. Flexor carpi radialis tendinitis: I. Operative anatomy. J Bone Joint Surg 1994;76A:1009–1014.
13. Breitenseher MJ, Metz VM, Gilula LA, et al. Radiographically occult scaphoid fractures. Value of MR imaging in detection. Radiology 1997;203:245–250.
14. Cerezal L, Abuscal F, Canga A, et al. Usefulness of gadolinium-enhanced MR imaging in evaluation of the vascularity of scaphoid non-unions. AJR 2000;174:141–149.
15. Cerezal L, del Pinal F, Abascal F, et al. Imaging findings in ulnar-sided wrist impaction syndromes. Radiographics 2002;22:105–121.
16. Chien AJ, Jacobson JA, Martel W, et al. Focal radial styloid abnormality as a manifestation of de Quervain tenosynovitis. AJR 2001;177:1383–1386.
17. Clavero JA, Alomar X, Monill JM, et al. MR imaging of ligament and tendon injuries of the fingers. Radiographics 2002;22:237–256.
18. Connell DA, Koulouris G, Duncan A, et al. Contrast-enhanced MR angiography of the hand. Radiographics 2002;22:583–599.
19. Cook PA, Yu JS, Wiand W, et al. Suspected scaphoid fractures in skeletally immature patients: application of MRI. J Comput Assist Tomogr 1997;21(4):511–515.
20. Di Fiori JP, Mandelbaum BR. Wrist pain in a young gymnast: unusual radiographic findings and MRI evidence of growth plate injury. Med Sci Sport Exerc 1996;28:1453–1458.
21. Di Fiori JP, Puffer JC, Mandelbaum BR, et al. Distal radial growth plate injury and positive ulnar variance in non-elite gymnasts. Am J Sports Med 1997;25:763–768.
22. Di Marcangelo MT, Smith PA. Use of magnetic resonance imaging in common wrist disorders. J Am Osteopath Assoc 2000;10:228–231.
23. Drape J-L, Dubert T, Silbermann O, et al. Acute trauma of the extensor hood of the metacarpophalangeal joint: MR imaging. Radiology 1994;1992:469–476.
24. Drape J-L, de Eery ST-C, Silbermann-Hoffman O, et al. Closed ruptures of the flexor digitorum tendons: MRI evaluation. Skel Radiol 1998;27:617–624.
25. Ecklund K, Jaramillo D. Patterns of premature physeal arrest: MR imaging of 111 children. AJR 2002;178:967–972.
26. Erdoes LS, Brown WC. Ruptured ulnar artery pseudoaneurysm. Ann Vasc Surg 1995;9:394–396.
27. Eustace S, Denison W. Magnetic resonance imaging of acute orthopedic trauma to the upper extremity. Clin Radiol 1997;52:338–344.
28. Flickstein JL, Bertocci LA, Nunally RL, et al. Exercise enhanced MR imaging of variations in forearm muscle anatomy and use: importance of MR spectroscopy. AJR 1989;153:693–698.
29. Futami T, Foster BK, Morris LL, et al. Magnetic resonance imaging of growth plate injuries: the efficacy and indications for surgical procedures. Arch Orthop Trauma Surg 2000;120:390–396.
30. Gabel G, Bishop AT, Wood MB. Flexor carpi radialis tendinitis: I. Results of operative treatment. J Bone Joint Surg 1994;76A:1015–1018.
31. Gabel GJ. Gymnast wrist injuries. Clin Sports Med 1958;3:611–621.
32. Gabl M, Rangger C, Lutz M, et al. Disruption of the finger flexor pulley system in elite rock climbers. Am J Sports Med 1998;26:651–655.
33. Girgis WS, Epstein RE. Magnetic resonance imaging of the hand and wrist. Semin Roentgenol 2000;35:286–296.
34. Glajchen N, Schweitzer M. MR features of de Quervain's tenosynovitis of the wrist. Skel Radiol 1996;25:63–65.
35. Golimbu CN, Firooznia H, Melone CP, et al. Tears of the triangular fibrocartilage of the wrist. MR imaging. Radiology 1989;173:731–733.
36. Grampp S, Henk CB, Mostbeck GH. Overuse edema in the bone marrow of the hand: demonstration with MRI. J Comput Assist Tomogr 1998;22:25–27.
37. Haims AH, Schweitzer ME, Morrison WB, et al. Limitations of MR imaging in the diagnosis of peripheral tears of the triangular fibrocartilage of the wrist. AJR 2002;178:419–422.
38. Harper MT, Chandnani VP, Spaeth J, et al. Gamekeeper thumb: diagnosis of ulnar collateral ligament injury using magnetic resonance imaging, magnetic resonance arthrography and stress radiography. J Magn Reson Imaging 1996;6:322–328.

39. Hauger O, Chung CB, Lektrakul N, et al. Pulley system in the fingers: normal anatomy and simulated lesions in cadavers at MR imaging, CT and US with and without contrast material distention of the tendon sheath. Radiology 2000;217:201–212.

40. Hergan K, Mittler C, Oser W. Ulnar collateral ligament: differentiation of displaced and non-displaced tears with US and MR imaging. Radiology 1995;194:65–71.

41. Huang HW, Strauch RJ. Extensor pollicis longus tenosynovitis: a case report and review of the literature. J Hand Surg 2000;25A:577–579.

42. Hunter JC, Escobedo EM, Wilson AJ, et al. MR imaging of clinically suspected scaphoid fractures. AJR 1997;168:1287–1293.

43. Imaeda T, Nakamura R, Shionoya K, et al. Ulnar impaction syndrome: MR image findings. Radiology 1996;201:495–500.

44. Johnstone DJ, Thorogood S, Smith WH, et al. A comparison of magnetic resonance imaging and arthroscopy in the investigation of chronic wrist pain. J Hand Surg 1997;22B:714–718.

45. Kato H, Nakamura R, Shionoya K, et al. Does high-resolution MR imaging have better accuracy than standard MR imaging for evaluation of the triangular fibrocartilage complex? J Hand Surg 2000;25(5):487–491.

46. Klauser A, Frauscher F, Bodner G, et al. Finger pulley injuries in extreme rock climbers: depiction with dynamic US. Radiology 2002;222:755–761.

47. Koskinen SK, Mattila KT, Alanen AM, et al. Stress fracture of the ulnar diaphysis in a recreational golfer. Clin J Sports Med 1997;7(1):63–65.

48. Kreitner K-F, Dieber C, Mäller L-P, et al. Hypothenar hammer syndrome caused by recreational sports activities and muscle anomaly in the wrist. Cardiovasc Intervent Radiol 1996;19:356–359.

49. Kumar BA, Tolat AR, Threepuraneni G, et al. The role of magnetic resonance imaging in late presentation of isolated injuries of the flexor digitorum profundus tendon in the finger. J Hand Surg 2000;25B:95–97.

50. Latshaw RF, Weidner WA. Ulnar artery aneurysms: angiographic considerations in two cases. AJR 1978;131:1093–1095.

51. Lohman M, Vasenius J, Kivisaari A, et al. MR imaging in chronic rupture of the ulnar collateral ligament of the thumb. Acta Radiol 2001;42:10–14.

52. Lohman M, Kivisaari A, Vehmas T, et al. MR imaging of suspected trauma of the wrist bones. Acta Radiol 1999;40:615–618.

53. Matlouk HS, Dzinierzynski WW, Erickson S, et al. Magnetic resonance imaging scanning in the diagnosis of zone II flexor tendon rupture. J Hand Surg 1996;21A:451–455.

54. Metz VM, Schratter M, Dock WI, et al. Age associated changes of the triangular fibrocartilage of the wrist: evaluation of diagnostic performance of MR imaging. Radiology 1992;184:217–220.

55. Munk PL, Lee MJ, Logan PM, et al. Scaphoid bone waist fractures, acute and chronic imaging with different techniques. AJR 1997;168:779–786.

56. Mussblicker H. Injuries to the carpal scaphoid in children. Acta Radiol 1961;56:361–368.

57. Nakamura R, Harie E, Imaeda T, et al. Criteria for diagnosing distal radioulnar joint subluxation by computed tomography. Skel Radiol 1996;25:649–653.

58. Nakamura T, Yabe Y, Horiuchi Y. Fat suppression magnetic resonance imaging of the triangular fibrocartilage complex. Comparison with spin-echo gradient echo pulse sequences and histology. J Hand Surg 1999;24B:22–26.

59. Oneson SR, Scales LM, Erickson SJ, et al. MR imaging of the painful wrist. Radiographics 1996;16:997–1008.

60. Oneson SR, Scales LM, Timins ME, et al. MR imaging interpretation of the Palmer Classification of triangular fibrocartilage complex lesions. Radiographics 1996;16:97–106.

61. Oneson SR, Timins ME, Scales LM, et al. MR imaging diagnosis of triangular fibrocartilage pathology with arthroscopic correlation. AJR 1997;168:1513–1518.

62. Palmer AK, Werner FW. The triangular fibrocartilage complex of the wrist: anatomy and function. J Hand Surg 1981;6A:153–162.

63. Palmer AK. Triangular fibrocartilage complex lesions. A classification. J Hand Surg 1989;14A:594–605.

64. Parellada JA, Balkissoon ARA, Hayes CW, et al. Bowstring injury of the flexor tendon pulley system: MR imaging. AJR 1996;167:347–349.

65. Patel MR, Moradia VJ, Bassini L, et al. Extensor indicis proprius syndrome: a case report. J Hand Surg 1996;21A:914–915.

66. Peh WCG, Gilula LA, Wilson AJ. Detection of occult wrist fractures by magnetic resonance imaging. Clin Radiol 1996;51:285–292.

67. Pfirrmann CWA, Theuman NH, Botte MJ, et al. MR imaging of the metacarpophalangeal joints of the fingers: II. Detection of simulated injuries in cadavers. Radiology 2002;222:447–452.

68. Plancer KD, Ho CP, Cofield SS, et al. Role of MR imaging in the management of "skier's thumb" injuries. Magn Reson Imaging Clin N Am 1999;7:73–84.

69. Potter HG, Asnis-Ernberg L, Werland AJ, et al. The utility of high-resolution magnetic resonance imaging in the evaluation of the triangular fibrocartilage complex of the wrist. J Bone Joint Surg 1997;79A:1675–1684.

70. Pretorius ES, Epstein RE, Dalinka MK. MR imaging of the wrist. Radiol Clin N Am 1997;35:145–161.

71. Rubin DA, Kneeland JB, Kitay GS, et al. Flexor tendon tears in the hand: use of MR imaging to diagnose the degree of injury in a cadaver model. AJR 1996;166:615–620.

72. Schweitzer ME, Natale P, Winalski CS, et al. Indirect wrist MR arthrography: the effects of passive versus active exercise. Skel Radiol 2000;29:10–14.

73. Saitoh S, Hata Y, Murakami N, et al. Scaphoid non-union and flexor pollicis longus tendon rupture. J Hand Surg 1999;24A:1211–1219.

74. Scheck RJ, Kubitzek C, Heisner R, et al. The scapholunate interosseous ligament in MR arthrography of the wrist: correlation with non-enhanced MRI and arthroscopy. Skel Radiol 1997;26:263–271.

75. Schimmerl-Metz SM, Metz VM, Totterman SMS, et al. Radiologic measurement of the scapholunate joint: implications of biologic variation in scapholunate joint morphology. J Hand Surg 1999;24A:1237–1244.

76. Seymour R, White PG. Magnetic resonance imaging of the painful wrist. Br J Radiol 1998;71:1323–1330.

77. Shionoya K, Nakamura R, Imaeda T, et al. Arthrography is superior to magnetic resonance imaging for diagnosing injuries to the triangular fibrocartilage. J Hand Surg 1998;23B:402–405.

78. Smith DK. Scapholunate interosseous ligament of the wrist: MR appearances in asymptomatic volunteers and arthrographically normal wrists. Radiology 1994;192:217–221.

79. Smith DK, Snearly WN. Lunotriquetral interosseous ligament of the wrist: MR appearances in asymptomatic volunteers and arthrographically normal wrists. Radiology 1994;191:199–202.

80. Smith DK. Dorsal carpal ligaments of the wrist: normal appearance on multiplanar reconstructions of three-dimensional Fourier transform MR images. AJR 1993;161:119–125.

81. Smith DK. Volar carpal ligaments of the wrist: normal appearance on multiplanar reconstructions of three-dimensional Fourier transform MR images. AJR 1993;161:353–357.

82. Sugimoto H, Shinozaki T, Oksawu T. Triangular fibrocartilage in asymptomatic volunteers: Investigation of abnormal MR signal intensity. Radiology 1994;191:193–197.

83. Swen WAA, Jacobs JWG, Hubach PCG, et al. Comparison of sonography and magnetic resonance imaging for the diagnosis of partial tears of finger extensor tendons in rheumatoid arthritis. Rheumatology 2000;39:55–62.

84. Tajiri Y, Nakamura K, Matsushita T, et al. A positioning device to allow rotation for cine-MRI of the distal radioulnar joint. Clin Radiol 1999;54:402–405.

85. Timins ME, Jahnke JP, Krah SE, et al. MR imaging of the major carpal stabilizing ligaments: normal anatomy and clinical examples. Radiographics 1995;14:575–587.

86. Timins ME, O'Connell SE, Erickson SJ, et al. MR imaging of the wrist: normal findings that might simulate disease. Radiographics 1996;16:987–995.

87. Totterman SMS, Miller R, Wasserman B, et al. Intrinsic and extrinsic carpal ligaments: evaluation with three-dimensional fourier transform MR imaging. AJR 1993;160:117–123.

88. Totterman SMS, Miller R. Scapholunate ligament: normal MR appearance on three-dimensional gradient-recalled-echo images. Radiology 1996;200:237–241.

89. Wottrich S, Lomaney LM, Demos TC, et al. Rupture of the ulnar collateral ligament of the first metacarpophalangeal joint ("gamekeeper's thumb"). Orthopedics 1998;21:1308–1312.

90. Yao L, Lee JK. Occult interosseous fracture: detection with MR imaging. Radiology 1988;167:749–751.

91. Zanetti M, Bram J, Hodler J. Triangular fibrocartilage and intercarpal ligaments of the wrist. Does MR arthrography improve the standard? J Magn Reson Imaging 1997;7:590–594.

92. Zanetti M, Hodler J, Gilula LA. Assessment of dorsal ventral intercalated segment instability configuration of the wrist. Reliability of MR images. Radiology 1998;206:339–345.

5

TUMORS AND TUMOR-LIKE CONDITIONS

THOMAS H. BERQUIST
MARK J. KRANSDORF

Benign tumors and tumor-like conditions in the hand and wrist occur much more frequently than malignant neoplasms (Tables 5-1 and 5-2).[3,6,13,19]

OSSEOUS LESIONS

Bone tumors in the hand and wrist are uncommon in comparison with the axial skeleton and lower extremities.[6,52] Benign tumors and tumor-like conditions occur more frequently than malignant neoplasms.[1,13,14,19,48–52,57] Routine radiographs or computed radiography images remain the primary screening technique for detection and characterization of osseous lesions. Computed tomography (CT) is a valuable technique for evaluating tumor matrix, subtle calcifications, and thin cortical bone. The image features of certain lesions, such as osteoid osteoma, are also characteristic on CT. Therefore, magnetic resonance imaging (MRI) of bone lesions is reserved for selected cases and staging of lesions (marrow, soft tissue, neurovascular involvement).[6]

Benign Osseous Lesions

Table 5-1 summarizes the most common benign and malignant bone lesions in the hand and wrist. Data vary depending on the series; however, the most common lesions are enchondroma, giant cell tumors, osteoid osteoma, aneurysmal bone cysts, exostosis, and osteochondromas.[13,19]

Enchondroma

Enchondromas are the most common benign bone tumor in the hand and wrist.[6,30] Up to 54% of these lesions involve the hand (Table 5-1).[13,19] Lesions may be isolated or multiple. Lesions usually develop during childhood but can be detected at any age.

Enchondromas are composed of lobules of hyaline cartilage and they are usually centrally located in the metaphysis.

Most are detected incidentally on routine radiographs or after pathologic fracture. When symptoms develop without fracture, malignant degeneration, though uncommon in the hand, should be considered.[6,19]

Radiographically (Fig. 5-1), enchondromas present as well-defined lucent lesions with areas of matrix calcification in some cases. Cortical expansion and thickening may also be evident.[13] Multiple enchondromas occur in Ollier's Disease and Maffucci's syndrome. Ollier's disease is a rare condition presenting with multiple enchondromas and shortening and deformity of the tabular bones (Fig. 5-2). The condition tends to be asymmetric or predominately involve one side of the body. Malignant transformation of enchondromas in Ollier's is more common than a solitary enchondroma. Maffucci's syndrome (Fig. 5-3) presents with multiple enchondromas and soft-tissue hemangiomas. Calcified phleboliths are commonly seen on routine radiographs. The hand is commonly involved. Unilateral involvement is noted in about 50% of patients. The risk for malignant degeneration of enchondromas in these patients is also increased.[13,19,45]

Magnetic resonance features of enchondroma have been described by Cohen et al.[18] Lobular high signal intensity was described on T2-weighted spin echo sequences. This was felt to be related to the higher water content of hyaline cartilage. The signal intensity on T1-weighted sequences is isointense in comparison with muscle. Areas of high signal intensity on T1-weighted sequences are usually related to marrow fat. Differentiation of benign from malignant is not consistent on MR images. Cortical destruction and soft-tissue involvement are useful features. Patterns of gadolinium enhancement are not specific.[4,5] MRI is rarely indicated in the hand and wrist due to the characteristic radiographic appearance.

Giant Cell Tumors

Giant cell tumors are locally aggressive lesions representing about 5% of benign bone tumors.[43] The lesions are most

TABLE 5-1. BONE TUMORS AND TUMOR-LIKE CONDITIONS IN THE HAND AND WRIST[13,19]

Lesions	No. of Total Cases	No. in Hand and Wrist
Benign		
Enchondroma[a]	726	392 (54%)
Giant cell tumor	1,301	156 (12%)
Osteoid osteoma	1,081	65 (6%)
Aneurysmal bone cyst	703	42 (6%)
Osteochondroma	727	28 (4%)
Osteoblastoma	225	9 (4%)
Chondromyxoid fibroma	112	4 (4%)
Exostosis[b]	1,177	37 (3%)
Fibrous dysplasia	347	12 (3%)
Benign vascular tumor	233	6 (2.5%)
Intraosseous ganglia	70	6 (8.5%)
Simple bone cyst	987	12 (1.2%)
Fibrous defect	505	2 (0.04%)
Chondroblastoma	294	1 (0.3%)
Histiocytosis	386	1 (0.02%)
Malignant		
Malignant vascular tumor	98	6 (6%)
Fibrosarcoma	391	1 (0.2%)
Chondrosarcoma	1,460	30 (2%)
Osteosarcoma		
High grade	2,956	14 (0.4%)
Central low grade	42	1 (2.4%)
Parosteal	157	1 (0.6%)
Periosteal	37	1 (2.7%)
Malignant fibrous histiocytoma	255	8 (3%)
Ewing's sarcoma	2,062	12 (0.5%)
Metastasis	5,680	29 (0.5%)
Myeloma	1,064	2 (0.2%)
Lymphoma	834	6 (0.7%)

[a]Does not include Ollier's disease or Maffucci's syndrome.
[b]Does not include multiple hereditary exostosis.

common after age 20 (20 to 40 years). The lesion is more common in females than males. Of the 12% that involve the hand and wrist, almost 85% involve the wrist.[13]

Radiographs (Fig. 5-4) demonstrate a lytic lesion in the metaphysis extending to the subchondral bone. The margins may be well or poorly defined. Cortical expansion, thinning, and fracture are evident in 33% to 50% of cases.[39,43]

Magnetic resonance features are not specific; however, the presence of hemosiderin results in areas of decreased signal intensity on T2-weighted images can suggest the diagnosis.[4] Typically, the lesion has signal intensity similar to that of muscle on T1-weighted sequences. Signal intensity is inhomogeneous on T2-weighted sequences with areas of high signal intensity, intermediate intensity, and low intensity due to hemosiderin in 63% of cases.[4,6]

Osteoid Osteoma

Osteoid osteomas are common benign bone lesions accounting for 12% of benign bone tumors.[13,19,32,38,61] Though osteoid osteomas can occur at any skeletal location, about 50%

involve the femur and tibia.[61] Most are cortical and diaphyseal or metaphyseal.[13,61] About 6% (65/1081; see Table 5-1) involve the hand and wrist. In the hands lesions are most common in the metacarpals and proximal phalanges. The scaphoid is the most commonly affected carpal bone.[13]

Osteoid osteomas can occur in the elderly, but most are reported in patients between 10 and 20 years of age. Lesions are much more common in males than females (3:1). The classic presenting complaint is pain at night. Pain is typically present from weeks to years, and 75% of patients report improvement following the use of salicylates.[61]

Edeiken divided osteoid osteomas into three categories.[27]

1. *Cortical osteoid osteomas.* This is the most common type, presenting with fusiform cortical thickening radiographically. The shift of the femur or tibia is most commonly involved. There is a characteristic lucent nidus that may contain mineralized material. In the small bones of the hand, periosteal reaction and marked swelling may mimic infection.
2. *Cancellous (medullary) osteoid osteoma.* These lesions are most common in the femoral neck, hands, and feet. Osteosclerosis is less extensive and may be some distance from the nidus. Lesions may be partially or completely calcified and surrounded by a lucent zone. Clear identification of the nidus is essential as it must be removed for cure.[13,61] The lack of sclerosis may make nidus localization more difficult.[19,61]

TABLE 5-2. SOFT-TISSUE TUMORS AND TUMOR-LIKE CONDITIONS IN THE HAND AND WRIST[12–14,37]

Lesions	No. of Total Cases	No. in Hand and Wrist
Benign		
Ganglion cyst	—	—
Pigmented villonodular synovitis (GCT tendon sheath)	410	180 (44%)
Hemangioma	443	53 (12%)
Lipoma	402	24 (6%)
Glomus tumor	52	27 (52%)
Neurofibroma	85	10 (12%)
Nodular fasciitis	19	2 (11%)
Myxoma	49	1 (2%)
Periosteal pseudotumor	182	20 (11%)
Malignant		
Synovial sarcoma	229	19 (8%)
Fibrosarcoma	311	13 (4%)
Malignant fibrosis histiocytoma	381	7 (.2%)
Rhabdomyosarcoma	91	3 (3.2%)
Leiomyosarcoma	70	1 (1.4%)
Malignant peripheral nerve sheath tumor	94	4 (4.2%)
Epithelioid sarcoma	31	10 (32%)
Liposarcoma	307	1 (.03%)
Extraskeletal chondrosarcoma	28	5 (18%)

GCT, giant cell tumor.

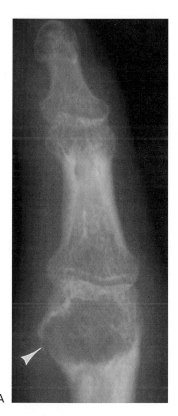

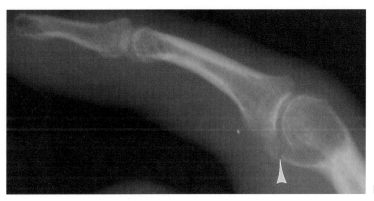

FIGURE 5-1. Posteroanterior **(A)** and lateral **(B)** radiographs of an enchondroma in the distal aspect of the proximal phalanx. There is a pathologic fracture *(arrowhead)* that resulted in its detection.

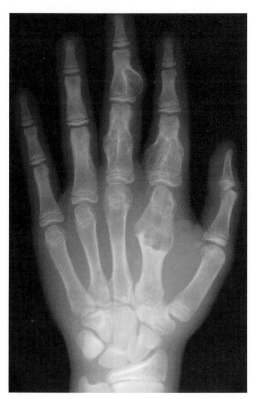

FIGURE 5-2. Posteroanterior radiograph demonstrating multiple phalangeal and metacarpal enchondromas in a patient with Ollier's disease.

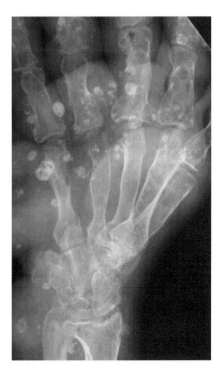

FIGURE 5-3. Oblique radiograph of the hand and wrist with multiple phleboliths and enchondromas due to Maffucci's syndrome.

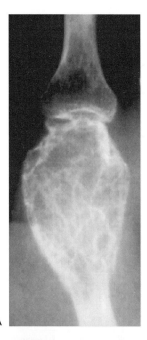

A

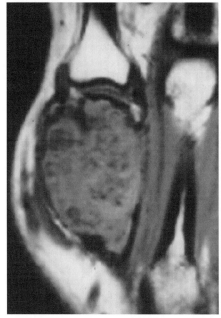

B

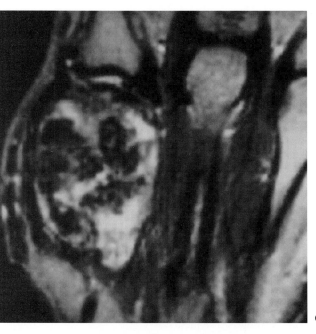

C

FIGURE 5-4. Giant cell tumor. **A:** Radiograph of the second metacarpal demonstrates a lytic, trabeculated expanding lesion. **B:** T1-weighted MR image shows a muscle density lesion with foci of low intensity. **C:** T2-weighted image shows large areas of low intensity due to hemosiderin.

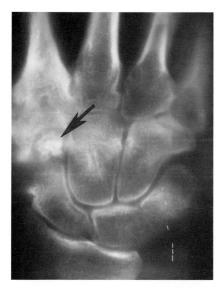

FIGURE 5-5. Osteoid osteoma. Tomogram of the wrist demonstrates a sclerotic focus in the trapezoid *(arrow)*. (Courtesy of Richard Berger, M.D., Department of Orthopedics, Mayo Clinic, Rochester, MN.)

3. *Subperiosteal osteoid osteoma.* This is the least common type of lesion. This lesion occurs in the femoral neck, hands, and feet. There is no reactive sclerosis. These lesions are most common in intra- or juxta-articular locations. In the hand, patients typically present with a soft-tissue mass.[27]

Computed tomography is the technique of choice for diagnosis of osteoid osteoma.[5] The nidus of a cortical or cancellous osteoid osteoma is a well-defined lucent area with variable surrounding sclerosis.

The MR appearance of osteoid osteomas (Fig. 5-5) has become more clearly described in recent years.[6] On T1-weighted images, the nidus is low signal intensity with low-intensity osseous edema. The nidus may be high signal intensity on T2-weighted sequences with surrounding marrow edema and synovial or soft-tissue inflammation. When there is significant calcification in the nidus, the signal intensity may be low on T2-weighted sequences.[6]

Aneurysmal Bone Cyst

Aneurysmal bone cysts are most commonly seen in patients 5 to 20 years of age. More than 50% of lesions occur in the long bones and up to 30% involve the spine. Six percent (Table 5-1) involve the hand and wrist.[13,19] Lesions may be multifocal, especially in the spine.[62]

Aneurysmal bone cysts are blood-filled structures with cavernous spaces separated by fibroblasts, osteoid, and woven bone.[20,44] Preexisting lesions are not uncommon (Fig. 5-6).[9]

Radiographs typically demonstrate an eccentric lytic lesion with thinning of the cortex and bony expansion. Septa-

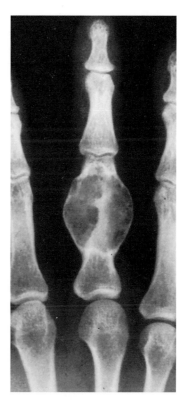

FIGURE 5-6. Aneurysmal bone cyst. Posteroanterior radiograph of the middle finger demonstrates a lytic expanding lesion of the proximal phalanx.

tions or trabeculated appearance is common (Fig. 5-6).[36,61] Faint-mineralized matrix may be evident in 13% to 16%.[6,62]

Magnetic resonance images demonstrate a well-defined, lobulated lesion with septations and multiple fluid-fluid levels.[6,36] Fluid-fluid levels are not specific for aneurysmal bone cyst but can be seen on T1- and T2-weighted sequences.[6,36] Similar features have been described in benign and malignant lesions.[6,36]

Osteochondroma

Osteochondroma is the most common benign bone tumor.[19,61] The lesion is thought to be related to a physeal growth defect or an abnormal focus of metaplastic cartilage due to trauma.[2] The most common locations are the femur, tibia, and humerus.[13,19] Only about 4% of solitary osteochondromas involve the hand and wrist.[13,19] Patients with hereditary multiple exostosis (autosomal dominant disorder) may also have hand and wrist involvement (Fig. 5-7).[13]

Most osteochondromas in the large tubular bones are asymptomatic. Those in the hand and wrist more often present with a palpable mass due to the superficial location of the osseous structures. Formation of an overlying bursa or malignant transformation is rare.[33]

Radiographs demonstrate a lesion originating near the growth plate region directed away from the epiphysis and

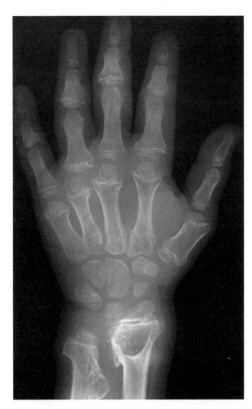

FIGURE 5-7. Osteochondromatosis. Posteroanterior radiograph demonstrates deformities of the epiphysis and metaphysis with multiple osteochondromas.

typically with marrow from the involved bone extending into the lesion. The appearance of the cartilaginous cap varies in the degree of mineralization.

Magnetic resonance imaging is not required for diagnosis of osteochondromas. However, if the patient is experiencing symptoms, or if malignant change is suspected, MRI can provide valuable information regarding the cartilage cap and surrounding soft tissues.[6] The cap is high intensity on T2-weighted sequences. The thickness of the cartilaginous cap is related to malignant degeneration, especially when it is greater than 2 to 3 cm.[6,61] Early enhancement on dynamic gadolinium-enhanced MR images along with curvilinear enhancement may be helpful in identifying chondrosarcomas.[6]

Other benign tumors and tumor-like conditions in the hand and wrist (Table 5-1) occur less frequently.[13,19,51,66] Therefore, they will not be discussed here.

Malignant Osseous Lesions

Primary and secondary osseous neoplasms in the hand and wrist are uncommon to rare depending on the histology.[6,17] In large series of lesions by Dahlin and Unni[19] and Campanacci[13], only 111 of 15,036 (Table 5-1) malignant

lesions involved the hand and wrist. With few exceptions, less than 1% of malignant bone lesions involve the hand and wrist. Malignant vascular tumors are uncommon in bone, but 6% are reported in the hand and wrist.[13,19,67] Three percent of malignant fibrous histiocytomas and 2% of chondrosarcomas involve the hand and wrist. Osteosarcomas and Ewing's sarcoma are reported but rare in the hand and wrist (Fig. 5-8).[53,54] When they occur, Ewing's sarcomas are more common in the metacarpals than phalanges.[53] Interosseous well-differentiated osteosarcomas are uncommon in any location but tend to be seen in the metacarpals or phalanges when they involve the hand. These lesions may be confused with fibrous dysplasia or enchondroma.[57]

To date, MR image features have not been useful for histologic differentiation of malignant bone lesions. Therefore, staging for marrow or cortical bone involvement and soft-tissue extension is the primary indication for MRI of suspected malignant osseous lesions.[1,6]

SOFT-TISSUE MASSES

Soft-tissue masses in the hand and wrist are not uncommon. The majority (Table 5-2) are benign.[6,12,14,30,65] The role of imaging, specifically MRI, is more significant when evaluating soft-tissue masses in the hand and wrist. Radiographs may demonstrate vascular calcifications (Fig. 5-3), localized soft-tissue masses and adjacent bone changes. CT remains useful in certain cases. However, the image quality achieved with new MR software and tissue contrast permits identification and, in certain cases, histologic characterization of soft-tissue masses.[6,7,12,14]

Ganglion Cysts

Ganglion cysts are the most common soft-tissue mass on the hand and wrist. Synovial herniation, tissue degeneration, repetitive trauma, and internal derangement have been suggested as possible etiologic factors.[6,28] The lesions most often occur over the dorsum of the wrist and distal interphalangeal joints of the hand.[6,28] Erosion of the dorsal lunate may occur. Twenty percent of wrist ganglia are volar arising between the flexor carpi radialis and abductor pollicis longus.[3] Associated tears in the triangular fibrocartilage complex are associated with ulnar ganglia. Radial ganglia may be associated with ligament tears or degeneration.[28] Ganglions may be cystic, filled with mucoid material, or complicated by hemorrhage. Most patients are 25 to 45 years of age, and there is a slight female predominance.[6,65]

Ganglia are usually 1 to 2.5 cm and may be simple or multiloculated. Ganglia may enlarge or resolve spontaneously. Nerve compression in the wrist is not uncommon.

Radiographs may reveal a focal soft-tissue prominence or dorsal erosion at the lunate.[3,6] Ultrasound demonstrates a

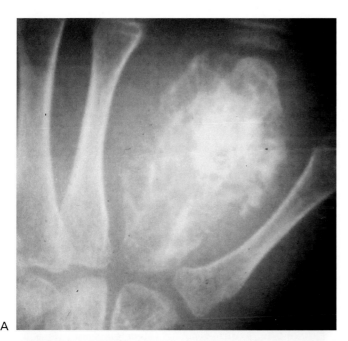

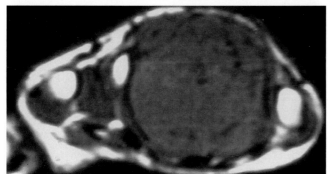

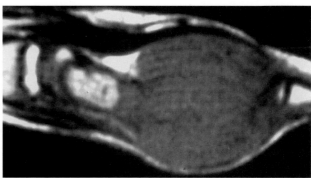

FIGURE 5-8. Ewing's sarcoma. **(A)** Radiograph of the hand demonstrates a destructive lesion with expansion and sclerosis of the fourth metacarpal. T1-weighted axial **(B)** and sagittal **(C)** images show a large mass with displacement of the adjacent metacarpals.

A

B

C

cystic lesion.[15] MRI demonstrates a well-defined lesion with high intensity on T2- and low intensity on T1-weighted sequences. Septations are not uncommon (Figs. 5-9 and 5-10).[6,8,25] Complicated (hemorrhage) ganglia or thick proteinaceous fluid may cause variation in signal intensity.[6] The effect of the mass on adjacent neurovascular structures is clearly demonstrated with MRI.[3,6]

Giant Cell Tumor of Tendon Sheath

Giant cell tumors of the tendon sheath are the second most common soft-tissue mass in the hand. Most patients are in their third or fourth decades, and, like ganglia, there is a slight female predominance.[42,63] There are local and diffuse forms of this condition. The local form (nodular tenosynovitis) presents as a nodular mass, typically in the hand or wrist (Fig. 5-11). The diffuse form typically occurs near a large joint and represents an extra-articular extension of pigmented villonodular synovitis (Fig. 5-12).[6,63,65]

In the hand and wrist, most patients present with a slowly growing mass, which is typically mobile and subcutaneous. The lesion is more common on the palmar surface of the hand and most often involves the first three fingers.[63] Lesions may be painful and multiple lesions, though unusual, can occur.[63] Malignant giant cell tumors of the tendon sheath have been reported, but they are rare.[16]

Radiographs demonstrate soft-tissue swelling or a focal mass (Fig. 5-13). Erosion of the adjacent metacarpals or phalanges occurs in 15%.[63] On MR images the lesion has signal intensity similar to that of muscle on T1-weighted images. Lesions may be high or low intensity and inhomogeneous on T2-weighted sequences. Areas of low signal intensity due to hemosiderin are typical of this lesion, similar to pigmented villonodular synovitis.[6] Fibroma of the tendon sheath may have a similar MR appearance.[6,63] Nonuniform enhancement is common after administration of intravenous contrast (see Figs. 5-12 and 5-13).[6]

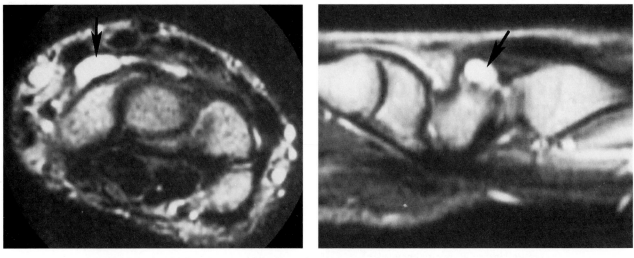

A B

FIGURE 5-9. Axial **(A)** and sagittal **(B)** T2-weighted images of a dorsal ganglion cyst *(arrow)* over the scaphoid.

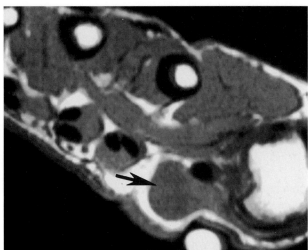

A

FIGURE 5-10. Axial T1-weighted **(A)**, proton density **(B)**, and T2-weighted **(C)** images of a septated *(open arrow)* ganglion cyst *(arrow)* adjacent to the flexor pollicis longus tendon.

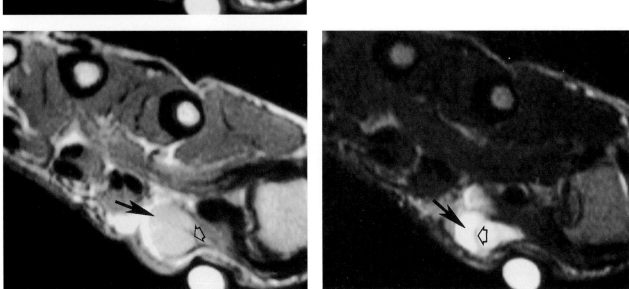

B C

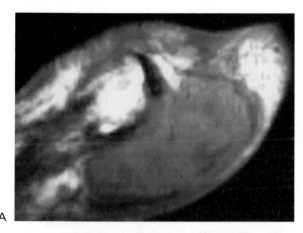 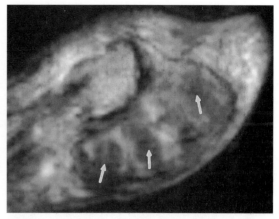

FIGURE 5-11. Sagittal T1-weighted **(A)** and T2-weighted **(B)** images of a giant cell tumor of the distal flexor tendon sheath. There are multiple areas of low signal intensity *(arrows)* on the T2-weighted image **(B)** due to hemosiderin.

Following resection, giant cell tumors recur in 50% of cases. Therefore, postoperative MR images serve as a baseline to improve accuracy for detection of recurrence (Fig. 5-14).[6]

Hemangiomas/Vascular Malformations

Hemangiomas are common, accounting for 7% of benign soft-tissue tumors.[59] Hemangiomas represent a spectrum of benign vascular lesions that resemble normal vessels histologically.[6,22,30,59,67] These lesions may also contain nonvascular elements such as fatty tissue, smooth muscle, fibrous tissue, and bone.[46]

Hemangiomas are usually classified according to vessel size as cavernous (large vessels) or capillary (small vessels). Lesions often have a mixed cavernous and capillary appearance. Nonvascular tissue is more often seen with cavernous hemangiomas.[11]

Vascular malformations are separated from hemangiomas in some classifications and institutions. Histologically and clinically they are not also clearly separated. We reserve the term vascular malformation in the context of arteriovenous hemangioma for lesions that clearly demonstrate venous and arterial components.[6]

Radiographs of patients with benign vascular lesions may demonstrate soft-tissue swelling or a mass and phleboliths

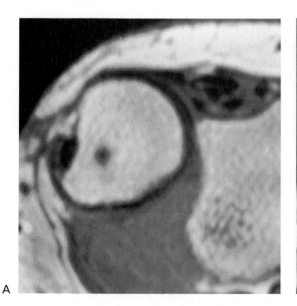 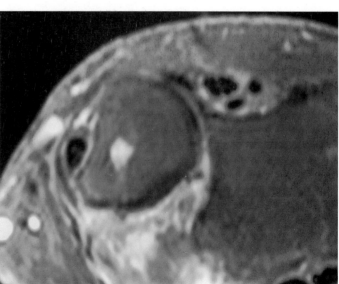

FIGURE 5-12. Pigmented villonodular synovitis extending from the distal radioulnar joint. Axial T1 **(A)** and contrast-enhanced fat-suppressed T1-weighted **(B)** images demonstrate the lesion with irregular enhancement.

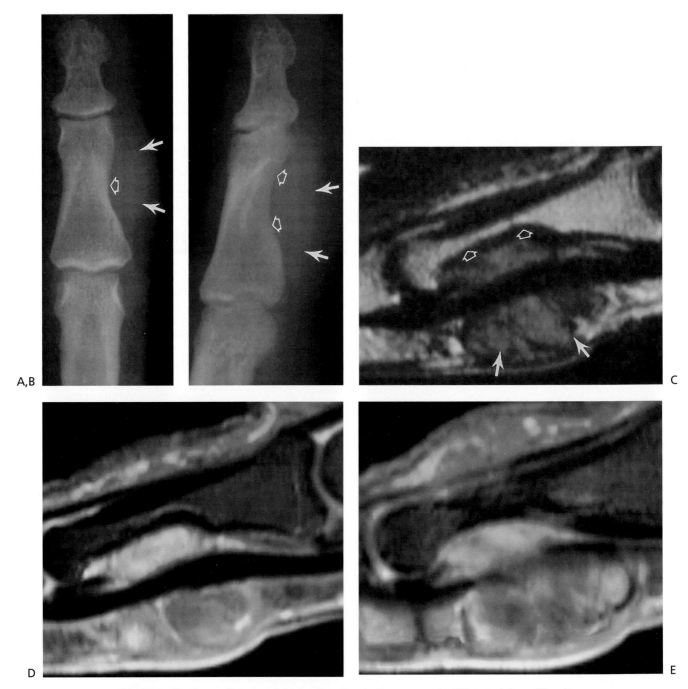

FIGURE 5-13. Giant cell tumor of the tendon sheath. Posteroanterior **(A)** and oblique **(B)** radiographs of the finger demonstrate a focal soft tissue mass *(arrows)* with bone erosion *(open arrows)*. T1-weighted image **(C)** demonstrates a large lobulated mass *(arrows)* around the flexor tendon with pressure erosion *(open arrows)* of the middle phalanx. Contrast-enhanced images **(D, E)** show inhomogeneous enhancement of the lesion.

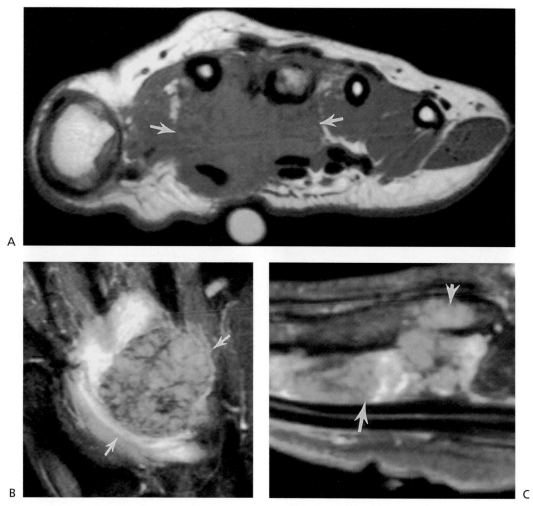

FIGURE 5-14. Recurrent giant cell tumor. T1-weighted axial **(A)** and contrast-enhanced fat-suppressed T1-weighted coronal **(B)** and sagittal **(C)** images demonstrate a large recurrent giant cell tumor *(arrows)*.

in the soft tissues. Phleboliths are most common in cavernous hemangiomas (30% to 50%). Conventional MR image features for hemangiomas are frequently characteristic. Serpiginous low signal intensity structures with intermixed fat signal are commonly seen on T1-weighted images (Fig. 5-15). Lesions are serpiginous or well defined with high signal intensity on T2-weighted sequences. Phleboliths are seen as round areas of low signal intensity.[6,11,30,59]

Hemangiomas and vascular malformations in the hand are not usually treated unless they interfere with growth in a child, are bleeding, decrease function, or become infected.[22] In this setting, conventional angiography or MR angiography is important to determine the extent and vascular supply to the lesion. MR angiography can be performed with conventional sequences (phase contrast or time-of-flight) or after intravenous gadolinium (Fig. 5-16).[22,59,67] Conventional T1- and T2-weighted images are typically obtained first;[6,67] 0.1 to 0.2 mmol/kg of gadolinium is injected, yielding three-dimensional gradient echo images (19/53/50°) (Fig. 5-17).

Subtraction can be accomplished by obtaining a precontrast mask image.[67]

Lipomas

Lipomas account for 5% of benign tumors in the hand and wrist.[31] Ganglion cysts, giant cell tumors of the tendon sheath, epidermoids, and hemangiomas account for the majority of the other benign lesions. Lipomas are composed of mature adipose tissue and are seen most commonly in middle-aged or elderly patients (>50 years of age). Lipomas may be superficial (subcutaneous) or deep. The former are difficult to separate from subcutaneous fat, except in the hand and wrist where there is less subcutaneous fat compared with the trunk or proximal extremities. Most lesions are solitary though multiple lesions are reported in 5% to 7%.[49]

Routine radiographs may be normal or demonstrate a fat density soft-tissue mass.[6,31] On MR images, the mass

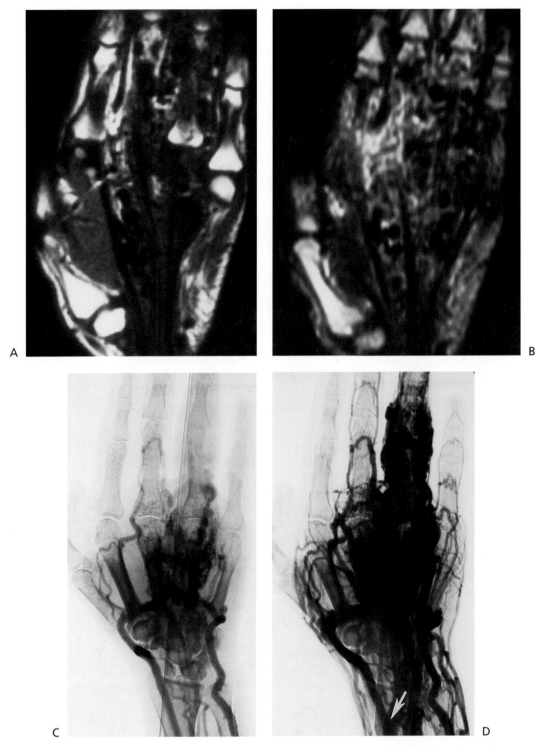

FIGURE 5-15. Arteriovenous hemangioma (arteriovenous malformation). Coronal T1 **(A)** and T2-weighted **(B)** images demonstrate multiple serpiginous flow voids. Early **(C)** and late **(D)** angiogram images show marked vascularity and early drainage veins *(arrow)*. (From Berquist TH. MRI of the musculoskeletal system, 4th ed. Philadelphia: Lippincott Williams & Wilkins, 2001:773–841.)

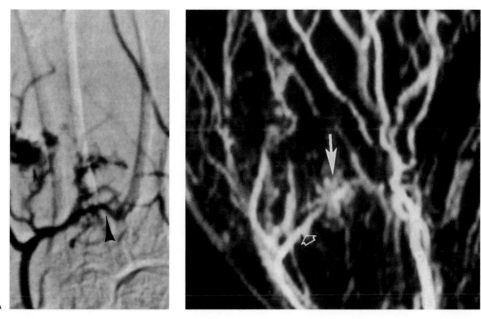

FIGURE 5-16. An 18-year-old with thenar vascular malformation. **A:** Conventional angiogram shows filling of the malformation via the deep palmar arch *(arrowhead).* **B:** Time-of-flight MR angiogram demonstrates the lesion *(arrow)* feeding vessel *(open arrow)* from the deep palmar arch. (From Disa JJ, Chung KC, Gellad FE, et al. Efficiency of magnetic resonance angiography in the evaluation of vascular malformations of the hand. Plast Reconstr Surg 1997;99:136–144.)

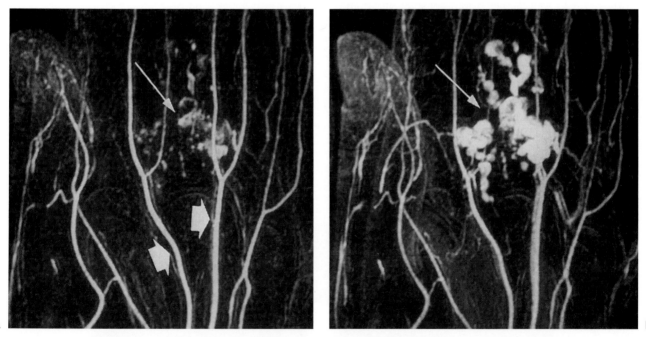

FIGURE 5-17. A 15-year-old boy with pulsatile mass volar side of the third digit. **A:** Contrast-enhanced angiogram shows the common and proper digital arteries to the second, third and fourth digits *(thick arrows).* The hemangioma fills at the base of the third digit *(thin arrow).* **B:** Second image obtained 45 seconds later shows the hemangioma *(thin arrow)* and its relationship to the proper digital vessels of the third digit. (From Connell DA, Koulouris G, Thorn DA, et al. Contrast enhanced MR angiography of the hand. Radiographics 2002;22:583–599.)

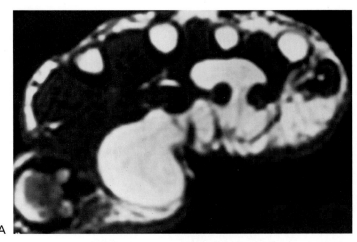
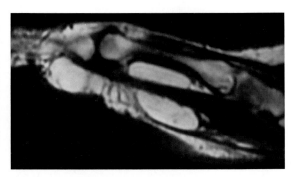

FIGURE 5-18. Axial **(A)** and sagittal **(B)** MR images demonstrating a large lobulated benign lipoma.

has fat signal intensity on T1- and T2-weighted sequences (Fig. 5-18). Though there may be well-defined septations or a lobulated appearance, there is no nonfat signal in simple benign lipomas.[6,23,31]

Intermuscular or intramuscular lipomas are deep and include variations (lipomas of the tendon sheath and neural fibrolipoma) common in the hand and wrist.[2,3,6,56] Fatty tissue in an intramuscular lipoma may infiltrate between muscle fibers giving a more irregular margin in comparison with the normally well-defined margins of a benign lipoma (Fig. 5-19).[6] This may also cause a more inhomogeneous MR appearance in this lesion.

Fatty tissue along a tendon can be seen in the hand and wrist (Fig. 5-18). Neural fibrolipomas typically present during early adulthood and involve the median nerve (80%). Patients present with a slowly enlarging wrist mass.[2,56] Patients may have pain, tenderness, and carpal tunnel syndrome (Fig. 5-20).[56] Up to 66% of patients have macrodactyly.[2,3]

Macrodystrophia lipomatosa is a rare localized form of gigantism that is present at birth. The condition is related to mesenchymal overgrowth in a single extremity and involves single or multiple (most commonly second and third) digits of the hand or foot. There is fatty tissue intermixed with fibrous strands. These features are easily appreciated on MR images (Fig. 5-21). Median nerve involvement (fibrolipoma) is not uncommon.[64] Clinically the differential diagnosis includes neurofibromatosis, hemangiomatosis, and Klippel-Trenaunay-Weber syndrome.[6,64]

Glomus Tumors

Glomus bodies are arteriovenous anastomoses responsible for thermo regulation. The unit consists of an afferent arteriole, tortuous arteriovenous anastomoses collecting veins and a neurovascular system that regulates flow through the anastomoses. Glomus bodies are present in the dermis throughout

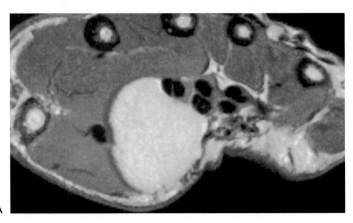
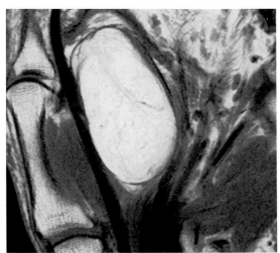

FIGURE 5-19. Axial **(A)** and coronal **(B)** T1-weighted images of a well-defined, slightly septated lipoma.

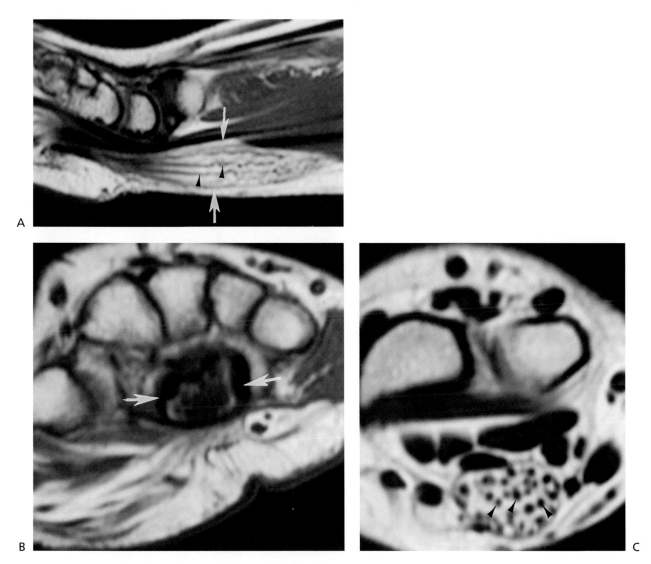

FIGURE 5-20. Fibrolipomatous hamartoma of the median nerve. Sagittal **(A)** and axial **(B, C)** T1-weighted images demonstrate a fatty lesion *(arrows)* in the region of the median nerve with low signal intensity strands of neural and fibrous tissue *(arrowheads).*

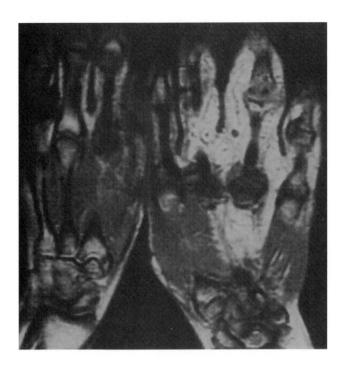

FIGURE 5-21. Macrodystrophia lipomatosa. Coronal T1-weighted images show fatty hypertrophy of the 3–5 digits. (From Wang YC, Jeng CM, Marcantonio DR, et al. Macrodystrophic lipomatosa. MR imaging in three patients. Clin Imaging 1997;21:323–327.)

the body, but they are most evident in the digits of the hand and foot.[60]

Glomus tumors are small (≤1 cm) hamartomas of the neuromyoarterial apparatus. They can occur anywhere in the body but most are located in the fingertips (75%), usu-ally beneath the fingernails.[10,12,21,52] Most lesions occur in patients 30 to 50 years of age. There is no sex predilection, although multiple lesions are more common in males.[21]

Clinical diagnosis is often difficult and may be delayed for up to 5 years.[10] These lesions account for only 1.2% to 5%

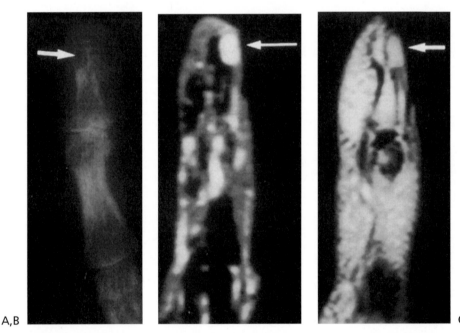

FIGURE 5-22. Glomus tumor. **(A)** Radiograph of the hand demonstrates a well-defined cystic lesion *(arrow)* on the ulnar side of the tuft of the fourth finger. Short TI inversion recovery (STIR) **(B)** and contrast-enhanced images **(C)** demonstrate the high signal intensity lesion *(arrow)*. (From Boudghene FP, Gouny P, Tassart M, et al. Sublingual glomus tumor. Combined use of MRI and three-dimensional contrast MR angiography. J Magn Reson Imaging 1998;8:1326–1328.)

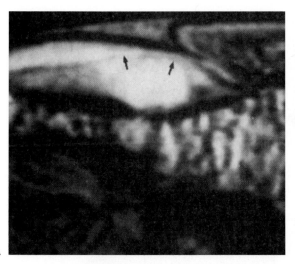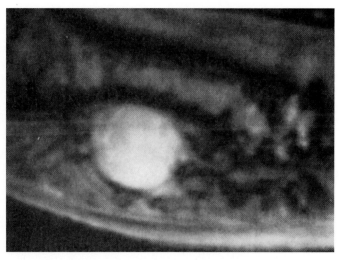

A · B

FIGURE 5-23. Glomus tumors. **A:** T2* gradient echo sagittal of a high signal intensity glomus tumor compressing the nail matrix *(arrows)* of the third finger. **B:** Sagittal postcontrast gradient echo image of a glomus tumor in the pulp of the fourth finger. (From Drape J-L, Idy-Peretti I, Goettmann S, et al. Standard and high resolution magnetic resonance imaging of glomus tumors of the toes and fingertips. J Am Acad Dermatol 1996;35:550–555.)

of all hand tumors.[21,25] Lesions may be painful, often exacerbated by changes in temperature.[55] Larger lesions may be palpable and tender when pressure is applied to the tumor.[10,21] Subungual lesions are more difficult to diagnose clinically. Unfortunately, 65% of hand lesions are subungual.[21] Lesions are usually solitary but multiple tumors are reported in 2.3%.[21] Detection and accurate localization is critical as complete resection is necessary to relieve symptoms.[10,21,25]

Radiographs demonstrate smooth bone erosions adjacent to the lesion in 22% to 60% of cases (Fig. 5-22A).[10,12,21,25,55] Ultrasound can identify lesions as small as 3 mm.[10] Improved spatial resolution with new surface coils has increased the role of MRI and MR angiography for detection and characteriza-

tion of glomus tumors.[10,21] Lesions are well defined and intermediate or low intensity on T1-weighted images and homogeneous high intensity on T2-weighted and STIR images (Fig. 5-22B, C). Lesions enhance uniformly after intravenous gadolinium injection (Figs. 5-22C and 5-23).[21,55] MR angiography can be performed using intravenous gadolinium and three-dimensional gradient echo sequences (5/2, FA 40°, one acquisition, 1-mm sections, and a 3-cm field of view). Gadolinium is injected (0.2 mmol/kg) at 2 mL/sec and flushed with 20 mL of saline with no scan delay (Fig. 5-24).[10]

The treatment for glomus tumors is surgical resection. Recurrence is common (5% to 50%).[60] In the postoperative

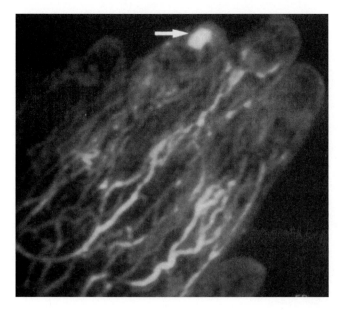

FIGURE 5-24. MR angiogram demonstrating a small glomus tumor in the ulnar side of the fourth distal tuft *(arrow)*. (From Boudghene FP, Gouny P, Tassart M, et al. Sublingual glomus tumor. Combined use of MRI and three-dimensional contrast MR angiography. J Magn Reson Imaging 1998;8:1326–1328.)

setting, MRI is useful to differentiate scar from tumor recurrence. Theumann et al.[60] reported MRI features of recurrent glomus tumors. Features were similar to those in preoperative studies described above in 54% of cases. In 33% (8 of 24), the signal intensity was low or isointense to subcartilaginous tissue. Slight enhancement of the contrast in 25% (6 of 24) was noted. Tumor margins were typically well defined, but irregular margins were evident in 38%.

Mucoid Cysts

Mucoid cysts have been provided with a number of terms including epidermoid cysts, dorsal cysts, synovial cysts, and myxomatous cysts.[24] Most are seen in elderly patients (mean age 63, range 40 to 70 years of age). There is frequently a history of trauma.[52] Lesions are most often located on the dorsal aspect of the fingers between the nail and distal interphalangeal joint.[24] Recurrence following resection is common.[52] Drape et al.[24] categorized cysts into three types: cysts in the proximal nail fold (48%), multiple flat cysts in the proximal nail fold (22%), and subungual cysts (30%).

Cysts in the proximal nail fold may be diagnosed clinically. There is frequently associated osteoarthritis and a pedicle leading to the joint. If the pedicle is not resected, recurrence is common.[24] Multiple flat cysts are more difficult to diagnose clinically but may be appreciated on ultrasound or MR images. These cysts are not associated with the joint. Subungual cysts are difficult to diagnose clinically. Bone erosion with subungual mucoid cysts is unusual (14%) in comparison with the above lesions, such as glomus tumors.[24,52]

Magnetic resonance images demonstrate well-defined high signal intensity lesions on T2-weighted sequences (Fig. 5-25). Intracystic septations were noted in 39%.[24] Using multiple image planes, joint communication is easily demonstrated in cysts proximal to the nail fold.[24]

Epidermoids

Epidermoid tumors are typically posttraumatic. Lesions are located in the distal phalangeal region and vary in size from 1 to 20 mm. Pain is a common presenting symptom. Lesions appear as well-defined lucent zones on radiographs. Bone erosion may also be evident.[24] On MR images, lesions have inhomogeneous signal intensity on T2-weighted images that may differentiate this lesion from a mucoid cyst. Lesions are low intensity on T1-weighted sequences.[24,52]

Benign Neural Lesions

Fibrolipoma of the median nerve was described above. Benign nerve sheath tumors (neurofibroma and schwannoma) and mucoid cysts in the nerve also occur in the hand and wrist.[3,29,47,65] Patients present with soft-tissue mass and/or signs of nerve compression.[3,6,29] Schwannomas present with a fusiform mass and more commonly affect the ulnar nerve.[3] Benign nerve sheath tumors are isointense with muscle on T1-weighted sequences (Fig. 5-26).[3,6] There are two useful MRI features on T2-weighted sequences. The "split fat" sign is seen when a peripheral rim of fat signal intensity surrounds the lesion. The target sign, seen with neurofibromas, is a low central region with high peripheral signal intensity on T2-weighted sequences. This corresponds to central fibrosis and surrounding myxomatosis tissue.[3,6]

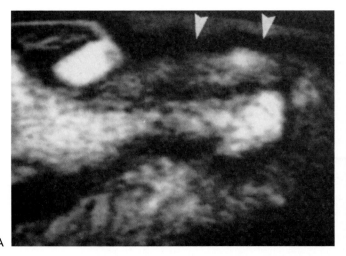

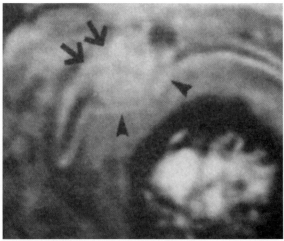

FIGURE 5-25. Mucoid cyst. **A:** Sagittal T2-weighted image demonstrates a well-defined high signal intensity 4-mm cyst in the proximal nail fold with distal nail atrophy *(arrowheads)*. **B:** Axial three-dimensional gradient recalled echo image shows the slightly hyperintense cyst deep to the lateral groove with compression of the proximal *(arrows)* and distal *(arrowheads)* nail matrix. The cyst healed after injection of sclerosing solution. (From Drape J-L, Idy-Peretti I, Goettmann S, et al. MR imaging of digital mucoid cysts. Radiology 1996;200:531–536.)

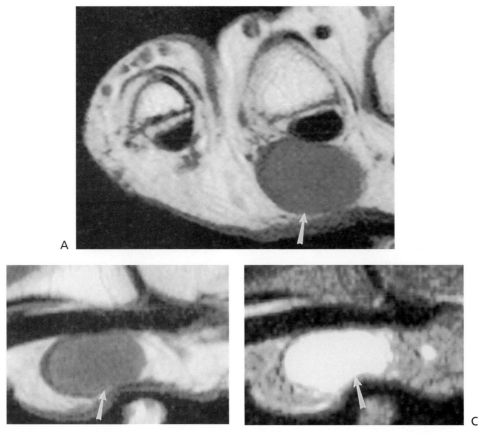

FIGURE 5-26. Benign peripheral nerve sheath tumor. T1-weighted axial **(A)** and sagittal **(B)** images demonstrate a well-defined low-intensity lesion *(arrow)*. Sagittal T2-weighted image **(C)** demonstrates a uniformly high-intensity lesion *(arrow)* in the fourth finger.

Intraneural mucoid cysts are most often seen in elderly males. Patients present with nerve compression symptoms. Of 21 cases reported by Giele and LeViet[29], 16 involved the digital nerves in the hand and 3 in the ulnar nerve in Guyon's canal. Etiology is uncertain. Lesions are low intensity on T1- and high intensity on T2-weighted sequences.[29]

Other benign lesions (Fig. 5-27; Table 5-2) in the hand and wrist occur less frequently.[34,35]

Malignant Soft-Tissue Tumors

Malignant soft-tissue tumors in the hand and wrist are uncommon. Only 4% of all lesions listed in Table 5-2 involve

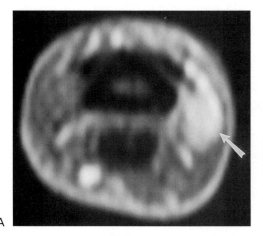

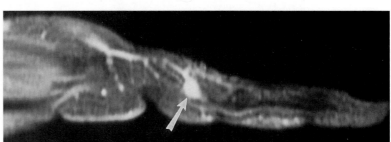

FIGURE 5-27. Benign fibrous histiocytoma. Axial **(A)** and sagittal **(B)** contrast-enhanced images demonstrate a high signal intensity lesion along the proximal phalanx *(arrow)*.

the hand and wrist.[13,65] Malignant fibrous histiocytoma is the most common malignant soft-tissue tumor in older adults (older than 45 years).[6,65] Only 0.2% involve the hand and wrist.[13,65] Capelastegui et al.[14] noted that only 3 of 134 soft-tissue masses in the hand and wrist were malignant (ma-

lignant fibrous histiocytoma, liposarcoma, rhabdomyosarcoma). Other malignant lesions (Table 5-2) involving the hand and wrist include synovial sarcoma (Fig. 5-28), fibrosarcoma, malignant peripheral nerve sheath tumors, epithelioid sarcoma, and extraskeletal chondrosarcomas.[12,13,40,65]

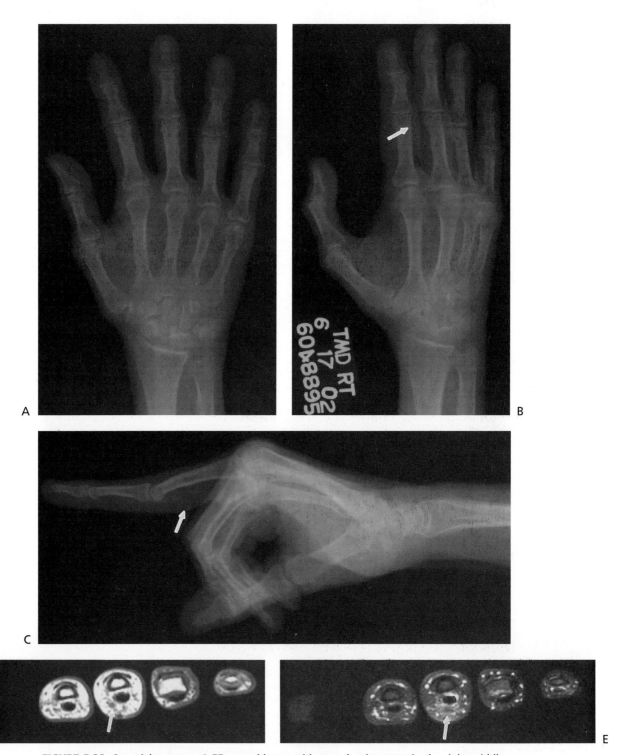

FIGURE 5-28. Synovial sarcoma. A 55-year-old man with an enlarging mass in the right middle finger. Posteroanterior **(A)**, oblique **(B)**, and lateral **(C)** radiographs demonstrate soft-tissue prominence *(arrow)* most obvious on the lateral view **(C)**. Axial T1- **(D)** and T2-weighted **(E)** images demonstrate an irregular mass *(arrow)* volar to the flexor tendon.

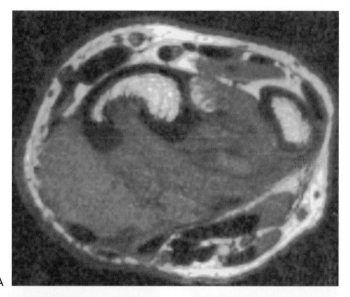

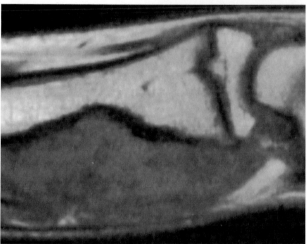
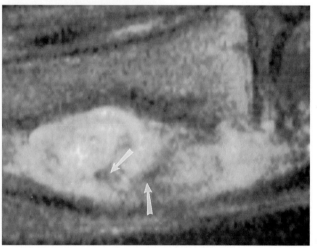

FIGURE 5-29. Recurrent desmoid tumor. Axial **(A)** and sagittal **(B)** T1-weighted images and sagittal T2-weighted image **(C)** show a poorly defined lesion with bone involvement. There are areas of low signal intensity *(arrows)* on the T2-weighted image **(C)**.

The MRI features of malignant soft-tissue masses are not specific (Fig. 5-28). Lesions are typically poorly marginated with low signal intensity on T1-weighted and inhomogeneous high signal intensity on T2-weighted sequences. Lesions show irregular enhancement after intravenous gadolinium. Necrotic areas do not enhance.[6]

Desmoid tumors are aggressive benign lesions that resemble malignant features on MR images. The presence of low signal intensity regions on T2-weighted sequences should suggest the diagnosis (Fig. 5-29).[6,37]

REFERENCES

1. Alam F, Schweitzer ME, Li X-X, et al. Frequency and spectrum of abnormalities in bone marrow of the wrist. MR image findings. Skel Radiol 1999;28:312–317.

2. Amadio PC, Reiman HM, Dobyns JH. Lipofibromatous hamartomas of nerve. J Hand Surg 1988;13A:67–75.

3. Anderson M, Kaplan PA, Dussault RG, et al. Magnetic resonance imaging of the wrist. Curr Probl Diagn Radiol 1998;Nov/Dec:189–226.

4. Aoki J, Tanakawa H, Ishii K, et al. MR findings indicative of hemosiderin in giant cell tumors of bone. Frequency, cause and diagnostic significance. AJR 1996;166:145–148.

5. Assorin J, Richardi G, Railhac JJ, et al. Osteoid osteoma. MR imaging vs. CT. Radiology 1994;191:217–223.

6. Berquist TH. MRI of the musculoskeletal system, 4th ed. Philadelphia: Lippincott Williams & Wilkins, 2001:773–841.

7. Binkovitz LA, Berquist TH, McLeod RA. Masses of the hand and wrist: detection and characterization using MR imaging. AJR 1989;154:223–236.

8. Blam O, Bundra R, Middleton W, et al. The occult dorsal ganglion: usefulness of magnetic resonance imaging and ultrasound in diagnosis. Am J Orthop 1998;27:107–110.

9. Bonokdarpour A, Levy WM, Aegerter E. Primary and secondary

aneurysmal bone cyst. A radiological study of 75 cases. Radiology 1978;126:75–83.

10. Boudghene FP, Gouny P, Tassart M, et al. Sublingual glomus tumor: combined use of MRI and three-dimensional contrast MR angiography. J Magn Reson Imaging 1998;8:1326–1328.

11. Buetow PC, Kransdorf MJ, Moser RP, et al. Radiologic appearance of intramuscular hemangioma with emphasis on MR appearance. AJR 1990;154:563–567.

12. Butler ED, Hamell JP, Seipel RS, et al. Tumors of the hand. A 10-year survey and report of 437 cases. Am J Surg 1960;100:293–302.

13. Campanacci M. Bone and soft tissue tumors. New York: Springer-Verlag, 1999.

14. Capelastegui A, Stinarsaga E, Fernandez-Cauton G, et al. Masses and pseudomasses of the hand and wrist: MR findings in 134 cases. Skel Radiol 1999;28:498–507.

15. Cardinal E, Buckwalter KA, Braunstein EM, et al. Occult dorsal carpal ganglion: comparison of US and MR imaging. Radiology 1994;193:259–262.

16. Carstens HP, Howell RS. Case report. Malignant giant cell tumor of tendon sheath. Virchows Arch 1979;382:237–243.

17. Cawte TG, Steiner GC, Beltran J, et al. Chondrosarcoma of the short tubular bones of the hands and feet. Skel Radiol 1998;27:625–632.

18. Cohen EK, Krusel HY, Frank TS, et al. Hyaline cartilage-origin bone and soft tissue neoplasms. MR appearance and histologic correlation. Radiology 1988;167:477–481.

19. Dahlin DC, Unni KK. Bone tumors: general aspects and data on 8542 cases, 4th ed. Springfield, IL: Charles C Thomas, 1986.

20. Dahlin DC, McLeod RA. Aneurysmal bone cyst and other non-neoplastic conditions. Skel Radiol 1982;8:243–250.

21. Dalrymple NC, Hayes J, Bessinger UJ, et al. MRI of multiple glomus tumors of the finger. Skel Radiol 1997;26:664–666.

22. Disa JJ, Chung KC, Gellad FE, et al. Efficiency of magnetic resonance angiography in the evaluation of vascular malformations of the hand. Plast Reconst Surg 1997;99:136–144.

23. Dooms GC, Hricak H, Sollitto RA, et al. Lipomatous tumors and tumors with fatty component: MR imaging potential and comparison of MR and CT results. Radiology 1985;157:479–483.

24. Drape J-L, Idy-Peretti I, Goettmann S, et al. MR imaging of digital mucoid cysts. Radiology 1996;299:531–536.

25. Drape J-L, Idy-Peretti I, Goettmann S, et al. Standard and high resolution magnetic resonance imaging of glomus tumors of toes and finger tips. J Am Acad Dermatol 1996;34:550–555.

26. Dreyfuss UY, Boome RS, Kranold DH. Synovial sarcoma of hand: a literature study. J Hand Surg 1986;11:471–472.

27. Edeiken J, DePalma AF, Hodes PJ. Osteoid osteoma (roentgenographic emphasis). Clin Orthop 1996;49:201–206.

28. El-Noulam KI, Schweitzer ME, Blasbalg R, et al. Is a subset of wrist ganglia the sequelae of internal derangements of the wrist joint? MR image findings. Radiology 1999;212:537–540.

29. Giele H, LeViet D. Intraneural mucoid cysts of the upper limb. J Hand Surg 1997;22B:805–809.

30. Girgis WS, Epstein RE. Magnetic resonance imaging of the hand and wrist. Semin Roentgenol 2000;35:286–296.

31. Goodman HJB, Richards AM, Klassen MF. Use of magnetic resonance imaging on a large lipoma of the hand. A case report. Aust N Z J Surg 1997;67:489–491.

32. Greenspan A. Benign bone forming lesions: osteoma, osteoid osteoma, osteoblastoma. Skel Radiol 1993;22:485–500.

33. Griffiths HG, Thompson RC, Galloway HR, et al. Bursitis in association with solitary osteochondromas presenting as mass lesions. Skel Radiol 1991;20:513–516.

34. Ha D-H, Jung W-H, Yoon C-S. Cutaneous hamartoma of the hand. MR image findings. Yonsei Med J 2000;41:147–149.

35. Höglund M, Muren C, Brattström G. A statistical model for ultrasound diagnosis of soft tissue tumors in the hand and forearm. Acta Radiol 1997;38:355–358.

36. Hudson TM. Fluid–fluid levels in aneurysmal bone cysts. A CT feature. AJR 1984;141:1001–1004.

37. Kasakowa Y, Okoda K, Hashimoto M, et al. Extra-abdominal desmoid tumor of the hand: a case report and review of the literature. Tokyo J Exp Med 1999;189:163–179.

38. Klan MH, Shankman S. Osteoid osteoma: radiologic and pathologic correlation. Skel Radiol 1992;21:23–31.

39. Levy WM, Miller AS, Bonakdupour A, et al. Aneurysmal bone cyst secondary to other lesions. A report of 57 cases. Am J Clin Pathol 1975;63:1–8.

40. Lim SC, Kim DC, Jeong YK, et al. malignant fibrous histiocytoma in a child's hand. Histopathology 1998;33:191–192.

41. Llauger J, Palmer J, Roson N, et al. Pigmented villonodular synovitis and giant cell tumors of the tendon sheath: radiologic and pathologic features. AJR 1999;172:1087–1901.

42. Maluf HM, DeYoung BR, Swanson PE, et al. Fibroma and giant cell tumor of the tendon sheath: a comparative and immune histologic study. Mod Pathol 1995;8:155–159.

43. Manaster BJ, Doyle AJ. Giant cell tumors of bone. Radiol Clin N Am 1993;21:299–323.

44. Mirowitz SA, Totty WG, Lee JKT. Characterization of musculoskeletal masses using dynamic Gd-DTPA enhanced spin-echo MRI. J Comput Assist Tomogr 1992;16:120–125.

45. Murphey MD, Flemming DJ, Boyea SR, et al. Enchondroma versus chondrosarcoma in the appendicular skeleton: differentiating features. Radiographics 1998;18:1213–1237.

46. Murphey MD, Fairbairn KJ, Parman LM, et al. Musculoskeletal angiomatous lesions: radiologic–pathologic correlation. Radiographics 1995;15:893–917.

47. Ogose A, HoHa T, Morita T, et al. Tumors of the peripheral nerves: correlation of symptoms, clinical signs, imaging features and histologic diagnosis. Skel Radiol 1999;28:123–128.

48. Oneson SR, Scales LM, Erickson SJ, et al. MR imaging of the painful wrist. Radiographics 1996;16:997–1008.

49. Osment LS. Cutaneous lipomas and lipomatosis. Surg Gynecol Obstet 1968;127:129–132.

50. Pahlos JM, Valdés JC, Gavilan F. Bilateral lunate intraosseous ganglia. Skel Radiol 1998;27:708–710.

51. Peh WCG, Ip WY, Wong LLS. Diagnosis of dorsal interosseous pseudotumors by magnetic resonance imaging. Australasian Radiol 1999;43:394–396.

52. Poznanski AK. The hand in radiologic diagnosis. Philadelphia: WB Saunders, 1984.

53. Saitoh S, Hatori M, Ehara S. Ewing's sarcoma of the middle finger in an infant. Orthopedics 2000;23:379–380.

54. Seymour R, White PG. Magnetic resonance imaging of the painful wrist. Br J Radiol 1998;71:1303–1330.

55. Shih TT-F, Sun J-S, Hou K-M, et al. Magnetic resonance imaging of glomus tumor in the hand. Int Orthop 1996;20:342–345.

56. Silverman TA, Enzinger FM. Fibrolipomatous hamartoma of nerve. A clinicopathologic analysis of 26 cases. Am J Surg Pathol 1985;9:7–14.

57. Sugano I, Tajina Y, Ishida Y, et al. Phalangeal interosseous well-differentiated osteosarcoma of the hand. Virchows Arch 1997;430:185–189.

58. Takhtani D, Saleeh SF, Chalker TL. General case of the day. Radiographics 1999;19:1394–1396.

59. Theumann NH, Bittoun J, Goettmann D, et al. Hemangiomas of the finger: MR imaging evaluation. Radiology 2001;218:841–847.

60. Theumann NH, Goettmann S, LeViet D, et al. Recurrent glomus tumors of fingertips: MR imaging evaluation. Radiology 2002;223:143–151.

61. Unni KK. Dahlin's bone tumors. General aspects and data on 11,087 cases. 5th ed. Philadelphia: Lippincott–Raven Publishers, 1996.

62. Vergel De Dios AM, Bond JR, Shives TC, et al. Aneurysmal bone cyst. A clinicopathologic study of 238 cases. Cancer 1992;69:2921–2931.

63. Ushijima M, Hashimoto H, Tsuneyoshi M, et al. Giant cell tumor of the tendon sheath (nodular tenosynovitis). A study of 207 cases to compare the large joint group with the common digit group. Cancer 1986;57:875–884.

64. Wang Y-C, Jeng C-M, Marcantonio DR, et al. Macrodystrophia lipomatosa: MR imaging in three patients. Clin Imaging 1997;21:323–327.

65. Weiss SW, Goldblum JR. Enzinger and Weiss' soft tissue tumors, 4th ed. St. Louis: Mosby, 2001.

66. Yamamoto T, Mizuno K. Chondromyxoid fibroma of the finger. Kobe J Med Sci 2000;46:29–32.

67. Yung BCK, Loki TKL, Chan YL. Angiomatosis of the hand demonstrated by contrast-enhanced magnetic resonance angiogram. Australasian Radiol 2000;44:198–200.

6

ARTHROPATHIES

THOMAS H. BERQUIST

Arthropathies and connective tissue disorders commonly involve the hands and wrists (Table 6-1).[3,4,33] Routine radiographs or computed radiography images provide valuable information for characterizing arthropathies and following treatment protocols. However, radiographs do not show early changes.[1,5,11,17] Also, direct evaluation of articular cartilage, synovium, and periarticular soft tissues is not easily accomplished. High-resolution magnetic resonance images with contrast enhancement provide a more accurate approach to evaluation and response to treatment compared with radiographs or radionuclide scans.[1,3,9,13,16] Magnetic resonance imaging (MRI) is also helpful in evaluating complications of arthroplasty procedures used in the management of arthropathies.

This section will review the arthropathies and connective tissue diseases affecting the hand and wrist, along with the role of MRI in detection and follow-up for patient response to therapy.

OSTEOARTHRITIS

Many factors contribute to development of osteoarthritis. Underlying disorders and joints involved may vary. Genetic factors, age, sex, obesity, trauma, and other conditions may all have a role in cartilage degeneration and underlying bone and soft-tissue changes. In general, this is a condition affecting the older population.[33]

Pathologic changes result in features noted on radiography (Fig. 6-1), ultrasonography, computed tomography (CT), and MRI. Cartilage fibrillation and surface erosions result in nonuniform joint space narrowing. Subchondral bony eburnation occurs due to bone formation and hypervascularity. Synovial fluid enters cartilage-bone defects resulting in subchondral cysts. Soft-tissue changes in the synovium, capsular distention with traction, and revascularization of remaining cartilage lead to osteophyte formation. Intra-articular osseous and cartilaginous loose bodies result from fragmentation of the articular surface.[33]

These findings on radiographs (Table 6-2) mirror signal intensity changes on MRI examinations (Fig. 6-2).[3,5]

EROSIVE OSTEOARTHRITIS

Erosive osteoarthritis is related to osteoarthritis but occurs primarily in postmenopausal women.[6] The distribution of joint involvement (Fig. 6-3) is similar to that of osteoarthritis; however, an inflammatory component results in erosions that can lead to ankylosis.[6,33] The changes give the joint a "seagull" appearance (Fig. 6-3). Erosions in erosive osteoarthritis are more central in comparison with marginal erosions seen with psoriatic arthritis.[6]

RHEUMATOID ARTHRITIS

Rheumatoid arthritis is the most common erosive inflammatory arthropathy and may progress to severe disability and deformity.[33,39,40] The condition may affect patients of all ages but is most common in individuals 25 to 55 years of age. Women are affected two to three times more frequently than men.[33] In early-stage disease, fatigue, weight loss, muscle stiffness, and malaise may mask the articular symptoms.[39] The disease may progress slowly with periods of remission or present with rapid onset and progressive disability and deformity.[33]

TABLE 6-1. HAND AND WRIST ARTHROPATHIES/ CONNECTIVE TISSUE DISEASES[6,33]

Osteoarthritis	Systemic lupus erythematosus
Erosive osteoarthritis	Scleroderma
Rheumatoid arthritis	Polymyositis/dermatomyositis
Juvenile chronic arthritis	Mixed connective tissue disease
Psoriatic arthritis	
Reiter's syndrome	
Ankylosing spondylitis	
Gout	
Calcium pyrophosphate dihydrate deposition disease	
Hemachromatosis	
Pigmented villonodular synovitis	
Multicentric reticulo- histiocytosis	

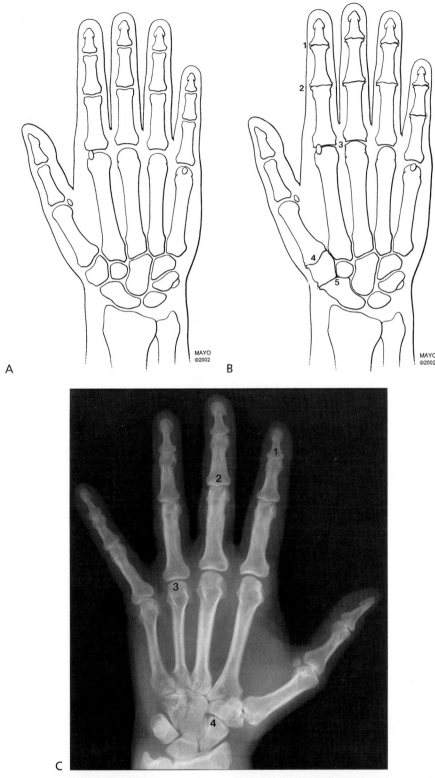

FIGURE 6-1. Osteoarthritis. **A:** Illustration of normal hand and wrist. **B:** Illustration of osteoarthritis with narrowed distal interphalangeal (DIP, 1) and proximal interphalangeal (PIP, 2) joints with marginal osteophytes. Narrowed metacarpophalangeal (MCP, 3) and first carpometacarpal (4) and scaphotrapeziotrapezoid (STT, 5) joints. **C:** Posteroanterior radiograph demonstrating joint space narrowing in the DIP (1), PIP (2), MCP (3), especially 3–5 and the STT (4) joints.

TABLE 6-2. OSTEOARTHRITIS: RADIOGRAPHIC FEATURES[6,33]

Bone density normal to increased
Nonuniform joint space narrowing
Osteophyte formation
Subchondral cysts
Symmetric bilateral distribution
Distribution: DIP and PIP joints > MCP joints, 1st CMC and
    STT joints.

DIP, distal interphalangeal; PIP, proximal interphalangeal; MCP, metacarpophalangeal; CMC, carpometacarpal; STT, scaphotrapeziotrapezoid.

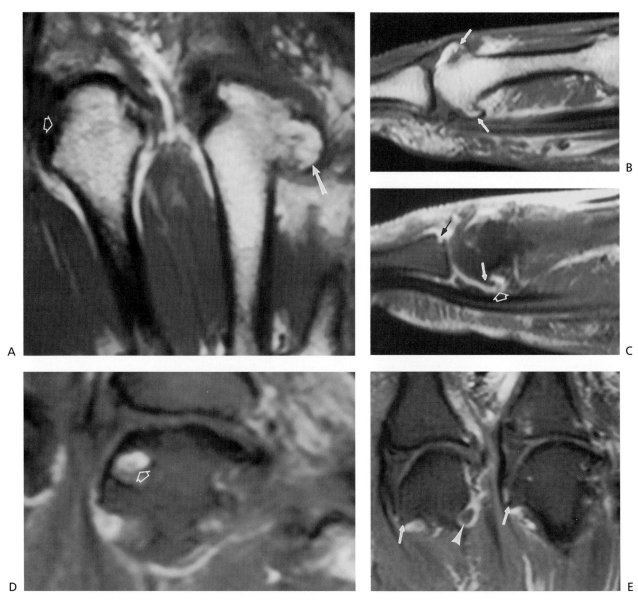

FIGURE 6-2. MR images of osteoarthritis. **A:** Coronal T1-weighted image demonstrating a prominent osteophyte *(arrow)* and bone sclerosis *(open arrow)*. **B, C:** Sagittal T1-weighted **(B)** and contrast-enhanced fat-suppressed T1-weighted image **(C)** demonstrating osteophytes *(arrows)*, synovial enhancement *(open arrow)*, and a small erosion in the dorsal middle phalanx *(black arrow)*. **D, E:** Coronal fat-suppressed T1-weighted contrast-enhanced images demonstrating osteophytes *(arrows)*, a geode *(open arrow)*, and a loose body *(arrowhead)*.

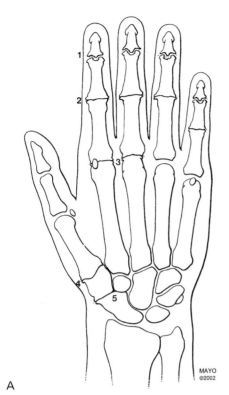 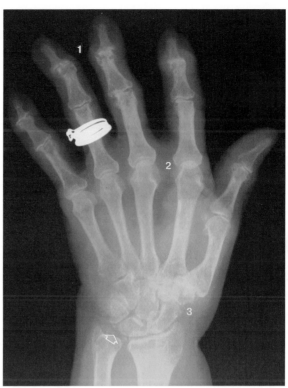

FIGURE 6-3. Erosive osteoarthritis. **A:** Illustration of change seen with erosive osteoarthritis. Note the "seagull" appearance in the second through fifth distal interphalangeal (DIP) joints (1) with more typical changes of osteoarthritis in the proximal interphalangeal (PIP) (2), metacarpophalangeal (MCP) (3), first carpometacarpal (4), and scaphotrapeziotrapezoid (STT) joints (5). **B:** Posteroanterior radiograph of the left hand demonstrating typical features in the DIP joints (1), narrowed MCP joints (2), and osteoarthritis at the thumb base and radial side of the wrist (3). There is also chondrocalcinosis in the wrist *(open arrow)*.

Clinical diagnosis may be established by characteristic symmetric polyarthropathy with morning stiffness, radiographic features of osteopenia, swelling, marginal erosions, and laboratory data demonstrating a positive rheumatoid factor and elevated erythrocyte sedimentation rate.[33,39,40]

Diagnosis in more atypical clinical presentations can be facilitated by using the American Rheumatism Association criteria, which are 91% to 94% sensitive and 89% specific when radiographic changes are present. Sensitivity and specificity are reduced to 87.5% and 62.1%, respectively, when there are no radiographic changes.[39]

Criteria include the following:

1. Morning stiffness about the joints lasting at least an hour
2. Soft-tissue swelling about three or more joints on physical examination
3. Swelling of the proximal interphalangeal (PIP), metacarpophalangeal (MCP), and wrist joints
4. Symmetric swelling
5. Rheumatoid nodules
6. Positive rheumatoid factor
7. Radiographic erosions in the hands and/or wrists with or without osteopenia

Rheumatoid arthritis is diagnosed when four or more criteria are met. Criteria 1 to 4 must be present for 6 weeks.[33,39,40]

Pathologic changes result in radiographic features described in Table 6-3. Rheumatoid arthritis affects synovial joints. The normal synovial joint (Fig. 6-4A) has articular cartilage with synovial membrane lining the joint capsule. At the margins, the synovial reflection abuts bone unprotected by articular cartilage (Fig. 6-4A).[33] In early

TABLE 6-3. RHEUMATOID ARTHRITIS: RADIOGRAPHIC FEATURES[6,33,39]

Periarticular soft-tissue swelling
Symmetric bilateral distribution
Juxta-articular osteopenia
Uniform joint space narrowing
Marginal erosions
Synovial cysts
Rheumatoid nodules
Distribution: PIP joints, MCP joints, with DIP joint sparing. Carpal joints, distal radioulnar joint, and ulnar styloid erosions.

PIP, proximal interphalangeal; MCP, metacarpophalangeal; DIP, distal interphalangeal.

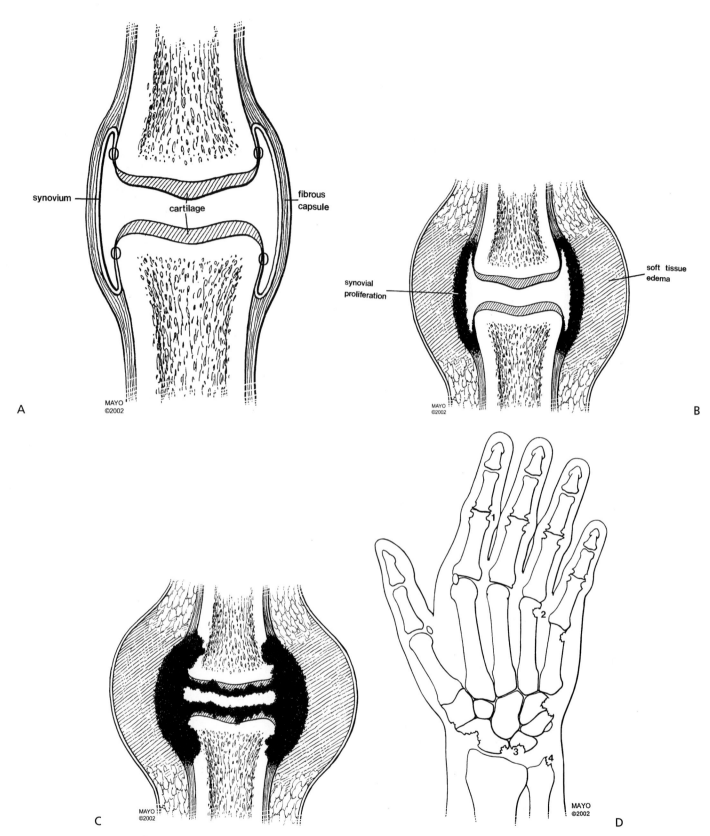

FIGURE 6-4. Pathologic synovial changes with rheumatoid arthritis. **A:** Normal synovial joint. There are marginal areas where synovial membrane abuts unprotected bone (0). **B:** Early changes with soft-tissue edema and synovial proliferation. **C:** Advanced changes with pannus formation and cartilage and marginal bone erosions. **D:** Advanced rheumatoid arthritis with marginal PIP joint erosions (1), narrowing and subluxation at the MCP joints, and erosions in the fourth and fifth metacarpal heads (2), carpal bones (3), and ulnar styloid (4).

rheumatoid arthritis there is edema and hyperemia with soft-tissue swelling and osteopenia. Synovial proliferation begins (Fig. 6-4B). With progression the proliferating inflamed synovium (pannus) extends across the articular cartilage resulting in surface erosion, which leads to joint space narrowing. Pannus in the marginal unprotected regions leads to bone erosions (Fig. 6-4C). Erosions in the hand most frequently involve the MCP, PIP, and interphalangeal joints of the thumb but spare the distal interphalangeal (DIP) joints.[33] In the wrist, erosions occur most frequently at the ulnar styloid, scaphoid waist, midcapitate, hamate–fifth metacarpal joint, first carpometacarpal joint, and radial styloid.[6] In advanced disease, subchondral cysts, subluxations and even ankylosis may occur (Fig. 6-4D).[6,33,39]

To date, radiographic features have been used to follow patients with rheumatoid arthritis (Fig. 6-5). The role of MRI for early diagnosis and monitoring response to therapy has increased in recent years (Fig. 6-6).[10,39,40,43] MR evaluation for arthropathies will be discussed more fully following the basic background sections of arthropathies affecting the hand and wrist.

JUVENILE CHRONIC ARTHRITIS

There are numerous articular disorders that affect children. Prior to reclassification most were grouped together in the category of juvenile rheumatoid arthritis.[6,35] Today these conditions are classified as juvenile chronic arthritis. A number of disorders are included in this classification. The exact category or condition may not be clear at initial presentation.[33] Juvenile chronic arthritis encompasses juvenile-onset (rheumatoid factor positive) rheumatoid arthritis, Still's disease (rheumatoid factor negative), juvenile-onset ankylosing spondylitis, psoriatic arthritis, arthritis associated with inflammatory bowel disease, and other miscellaneous arthropathies.[6]

Still's disease accounts for 70% of cases of juvenile chronic arthritis and usually occurs in young children (Fig. 6-7). Three patterns of disease have been described. The first is classic systemic disease with no articular involvement (rash, fever, pericarditis or myocarditis, adenopathy, and hepatosplenomegaly). Polyarthropathy with lesser systemic symptoms occurs in 20% of cases of juvenile chronic arthritis. Mono- or pauciarticular disease is evident in 30% to 70% of children with juvenile chronic arthritis.[6,33] Pauci- or monoarticular disease tends to involve the larger joints (knees, ankles, elbows), but the wrist is also commonly affected (Fig. 6-8).[33] All types of Still's disease tend to involve younger children (≤5 years of age), in comparison with seropositive rheumatoid arthritis or spondyloarthropathies (≥10 years of age).[33]

Juvenile-onset (seropositive) rheumatoid arthritis differs from the adult form of this condition in that periostitis is often present and joint spaces are preserved in the presence of marginal erosions (Fig. 6-7A).[6]

Patients with Still's disease have radiographic features that differ due to the rapidly growing phase of their osseous structures (Fig. 6-17). The hand is involved less frequently than the wrist, but when affected, the DIP, PIP, and MCP joints may be involved. Osteopenia and periarticular swelling are common (Fig. 6-8). Metadiaphyseal periostitis is evident in nearly one-fourth of patients.[6] Overgrowth of epiphyses and premature physeal fusion is common. Erosive disease tends to occur later with preservation of the joint spaces.[6,46]

PSORIATIC ARTHRITIS

Psoriatic arthritis has an age distribution similar to rheumatoid arthritis (25 to 55 years). The disorder is now frequently detected in children as well as adults.[33] Most patients have psoriatic skin disease for a long time prior to developing arthropathy, although joint disease may precede or occur simultaneously with the skin disease.[6,34] The incidence of arthropathy varies widely but most agree that joint involvement probably occurs in 2% to 6% of patients with psoriasis. The joints of the hands and feet are involved in up to 75% of patients with joint disease.[33,34]

Radiographic features of psoriatic arthritis may overlap with those of Reiter's ankylosing spondylitis and rheumatoid arthritis.[6] Table 6-4 summarizes radiographic features. The most helpful radiographic features are fusiform ("sausage digit") swelling, bone proliferation, and DIP joint involvement (Fig. 6-9). Bone proliferation is commonly seen adjacent to erosions and at tendon and ligament attachments. Brower[6] described three characteristic patterns. The first is DIP and PIP joint involvement with proximal sparing; the second involves all joints or three fingers; and the third pattern is similar to that for rheumatoid arthritis except for bone proliferation and distal joint involvement.[6]

REITER'S SYNDROME

Reiter's syndrome occurs most commonly in males 15 to 35 years of age. The condition is uncommon in the general population but more common in the military. It may follow sexual transmission or dysentery. In males, the triad of arthropathy, urethritis, and conjunctivitis is common. Females are much less frequently affected. In general, females present with Reiter's syndrome after dysentery (bacillus, amebic, or *Shigella*) and may have cystitis and conjunctivitis.[33]

The arthropathy most often involves the lower extremities in a bilateral asymmetric pattern. The knee, ankle, and foot are commonly involved (Table 6-5). The hand and wrist are not commonly involved, unlike psoriatic arthritis.[6] Fusiform soft-tissue swelling and osteopenia about the joints may be evident early on radiographs.[6] Bone density remains normal. Involvement of only one or two digits is common (Fig. 6-10).[6,33]

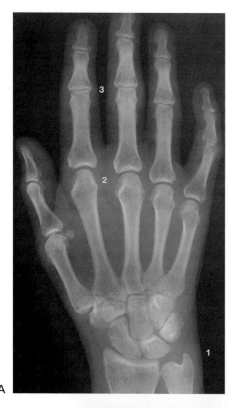

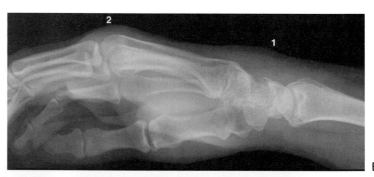

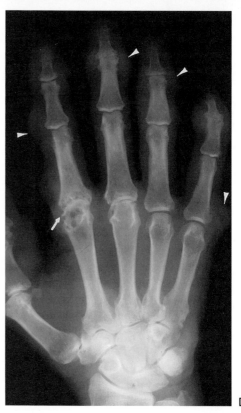

FIGURE 6-5. Radiographic features of rheumatoid arthritis. **A, B:** Early rheumatoid arthritis seen on anteroposterior **(A)** and lateral **(B)** radiographs with soft-tissue swelling in the wrist (1), metacarpophalangeal (MCP) joint swelling and synovitis (2), and proximal interphalangeal (PIP) joint (3) swelling. No bone erosions. **C:** Posteroanterior (PA) radiograph in more advanced disease with ulnar deviation of the second through fourth fingers (→) MCP erosions (1), and erosions in the lunate (2) and ulnar styloid (3). **D:** PA radiograph with advanced erosive changes in the second MCP joint *(arrow)* and multiple rheumatoid nodules *(arrowheads)*.

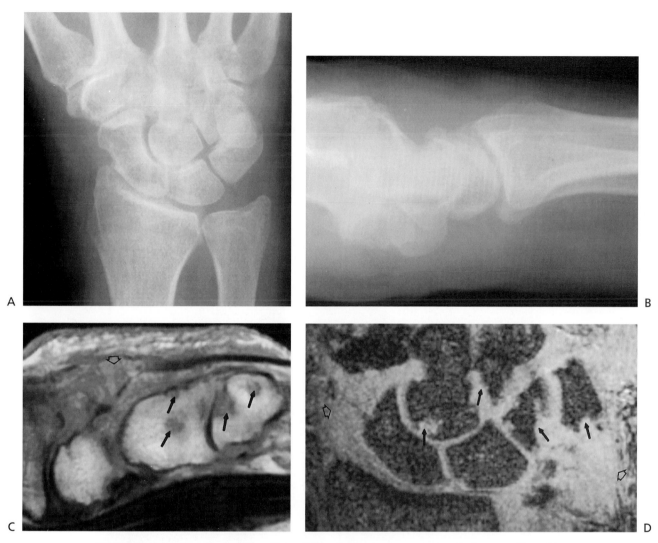

FIGURE 6-6. Posteroanterior **(A)** and lateral **(B)** radiographs demonstrate soft-tissue swelling with no erosions. Sagittal T1 **(C)** and coronal gradient recalled echo **(D)** MR images demonstrate erosions *(arrows)* and increased signal *(open arrows)* on image D due to synovitis. Synovitis is intermediate in signal intensity *(open arrow)* on the dorsal aspect of the T1-weighted image **(C)**.

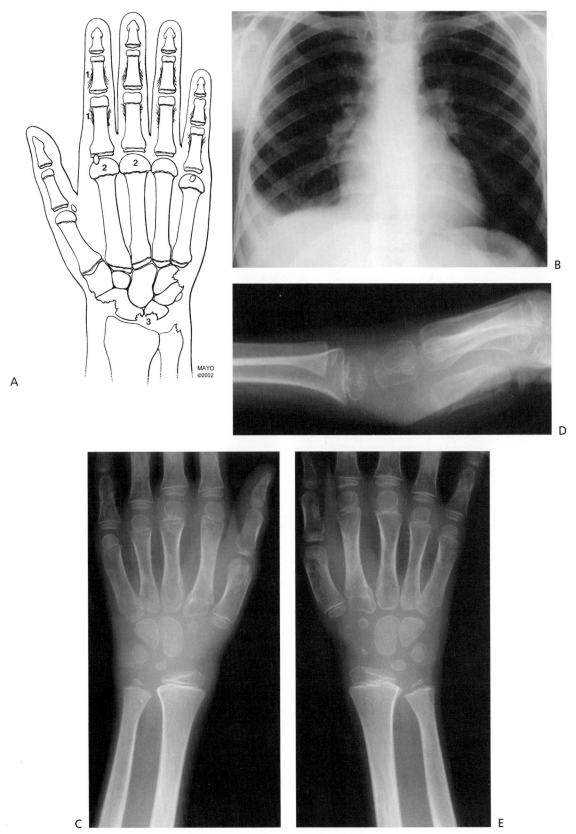

FIGURE 6-7. Juvenile chronic arthritis. **A:** Illustration demonstrating periostitis (1), preserved joint spaces, enlarged metacarpal heads (2), and carpal erosions (3). **B–F:** Still's disease. Chest radiograph **(B)** demonstrates a right pleural effusion. Posteroanterior and lateral radiographs of the left **(C, D)** and right **(E, F)** wrists demonstrate swelling and osteopenia. For a 7-year-old boy, the trapezium, trapezoid, scaphoid, and lunate are underdeveloped or partially resorbed.

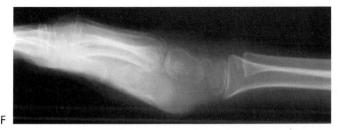

F

FIGURE 6-7. (*continued*)

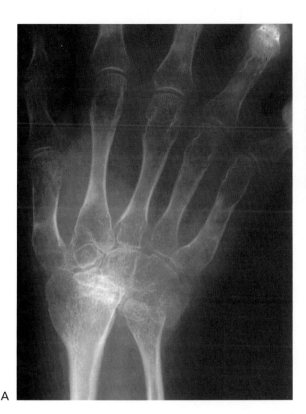

A

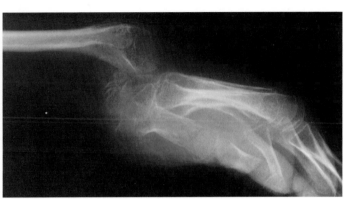

B

FIGURE 6-8. Juvenile chronic arthritis. Posteroanterior **(A)** and lateral **(B)** radiographs demonstrate marked osteopenia, carpal collapse, and volar dislocation at the wrist.

TABLE 6-4. PSORIATIC ARTHRITIS: RADIOGRAPHIC FEATURES[6,33]

Fusiform soft-tissue swelling ("sausage digit")
Normal bone density
Bone proliferation
Pencil-in-cup deformity
Erosions, marginal and central
Asymmetric bilateral distribution
Ankylosis
Distribution: Phalangeal joints with DIP most common. Carpal bones may be spared or be similar to rheumatoid arthritis.

DIP, distal interphalangeal.

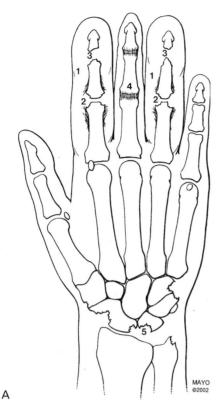

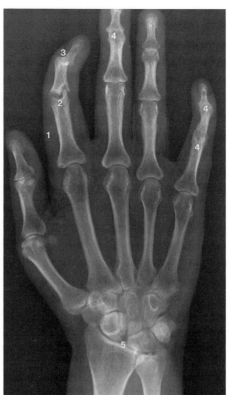

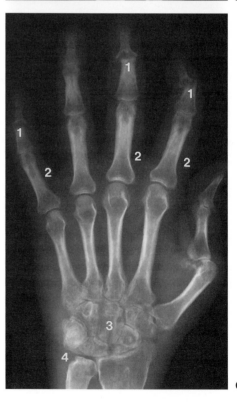

FIGURE 6-9. Psoriatic arthritis. **A:** Illustration demonstrating fusiform swelling ("sausage digit") (1) of the second and fourth fingers, periostitis with marginal erosions (2) [greater involvement at the distal interphalangeal, or DIP, joints (3)], ankylosis of the third DIP and proximal interphalangeal, or PIP, joints (4), and erosions in the wrist (5). **B:** Posteroanterior (PA) radiograph of the hand and wrist demonstrates fusiform swelling of the index finger (1) with PIP (2) erosions and DIP subluxation (3). There is ankylosis of the third and fifth DIP joints and fifth PIP joint (4). There is narrowing of joint spaces in the wrist with scapholunate erosions (5). **C:** PA radiograph of the right hand and wrist demonstrates erosions in the second, third, and fifth DIP joints (1) with fusiform swelling of the second, third, and, to a lesser degree, fifth fingers (2). There is swelling and joint space narrowing in the wrist (3) with an obvious ulnar styloid erosion (4).

TABLE 6-5. REITER'S SYNDROME: RADIOGRAPHIC FEATURES[6,33]

Fusiform soft-tissue swelling ("sausage digit")
Normal bone density
Bone proliferation
Marginal erosions
Uniform joint space narrowing
Bilateral asymmetric distribution
Distribution: Lower extremity predominates. PIP joints of hand more common than DIP or MCP. Carpal and ulnar styloid erosions.

PIP, proximal interphalangeal; DIP, distal interphalangeal; MCP, metacarpophalangeal.

TABLE 6-6. ANKYLOSING SPONDYLITIS: RADIOGRAPHIC FEATURES[6,33]

Normal bone mineral
Subchondral bone formation
Ankylosis
No subluxations
No subchondral cysts
Bilateral symmetric
Distribution: Sacroiliac joints and spine. Hands and wrists uncommon.

ANKYLOSING SPONDYLITIS

Patients with ankylosing spondylitis typically present with low back pain, stiffness, and limited motion. This condition involves 0.1% of the general population, with males outnumbering females 4–10:1.[33] Patients are typically 15 to 35 years of age. Ankylosing spondylitis involves the sacroiliac joints and spine; however, the peripheral skeleton is involved in 10% to 20% of patients.[6,33]

Radiographically (Table 6-6), enthesopathy, ankylosis, and symmetric sacroiliac joint involvement are distinguishing features. Bone mineral is normal.[6] In the hand and wrist, bone ankylosis and bone formation may be evident (Fig. 6-11).

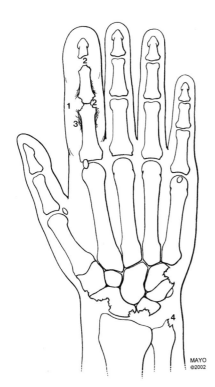

FIGURE 6-10. Reiter's syndrome. Illustration of radiograph features with fusiform swelling of the index finger (1), distal and proximal interphalangeal erosions (2), and periostitis (3). There are erosions in the wrist, including the ulnar styloid (4).

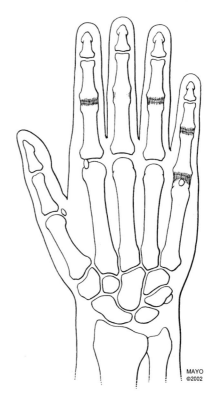

FIGURE 6-11. Ankylosing spondylitis. Illustration demonstrating varying degrees of ankylosis in the second through fifth proximal interphalangeal and fifth metacarpophalangeal joints.

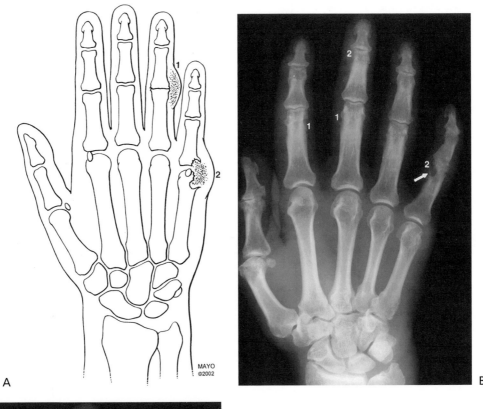

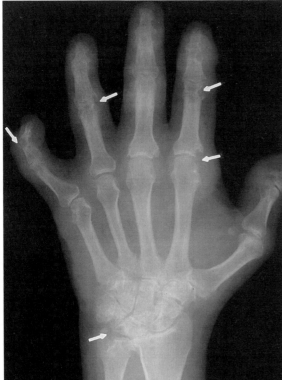

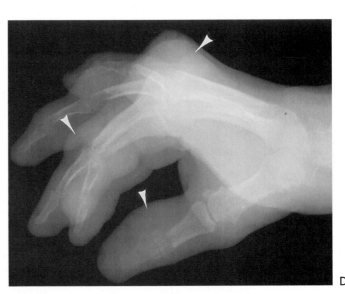

FIGURE 6-12. Gout. **A:** Illustration of soft-tissue tophus with calcification (1) and bone erosions with overhanging margins and soft-tissue changes (2). **B:** Posteroanterior (PA) radiograph demonstrating degenerative changes and bone proliferation (1) with erosions (2) most obvious at the fifth PIP with overhanging margins *(arrow)*. **C–F:** PA and lateral radiographs of the left **(C, D)** and right **(E, F)** hands and wrists with erosions *(arrows)* and numerous soft-tissue tophi *(arrowheads)*.

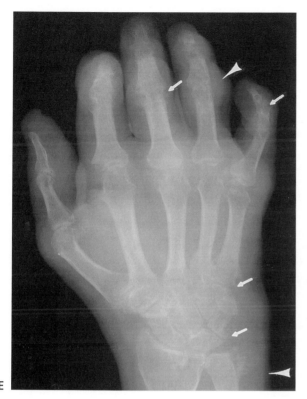

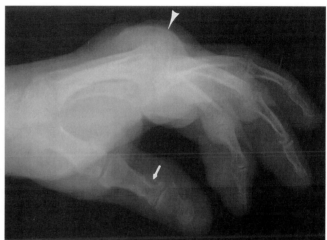

FIGURE 6-12. (*continued*)

GOUT

Gout may be primary (inborn error in uric acid metabolism) or secondary (other associated diseases). Secondary gout is not usually associated with radiographic changes.[6,33] Gout affects males more commonly than females (20:1). Females with gout are typically postmenopausal. Males typically present with their first symptoms in the fifth decade.[6]

Radiographic features (Fig. 6-12) are the result of chronic hyperuricemia and deposition of monosodium urate crystals in cartilage, bone, or soft tissues. Gout is typically monoarticular and more commonly involves the lower extremity, specifically the feet. Radiographic features (Table 6-7) are usually not evident for 6 to 8 years. Up to 45% of patients develop bone changes.[6] Radiographic changes occur based on the location of monosodium urate crystal deposition.

TABLE 6-7. GOUT: RADIOGRAPHIC FEATURES[6,33]

Normal bone mineral
Joint space preserved
Erosions with overhanging edge
Asymmetric involvement
Tophi
Distribution: Lower extremity > hand and wrist. DIP, PIP, MCP, and CMC joints of the hand. Carpal bones, distal radioulnar joint of the wrist.

DIP, distal interphalangeal; PIP, proximal interphalangeal; MCP, metacarpophalangeal; CMC, carpometacarpal.

Deposition in the soft tissues results in soft-tissue masses (tophi) (Fig. 6-12A, C–F), which frequently contain calcifications. Bone erosion is common with well-defined margins and over time remodels to form an overhanging edge (Fig. 6-12A-F).[6,33] The overhanging edge phenomenon may be seen in up to 40% of erosions. Bone mineral is typically normal in patients with gouty arthropathy.[6]

CALCIUM PYROPHOSPHATE DEPOSITION DISEASE

Calcium pyrophosphate deposition disease (CPPD) is a common arthropathy in the middle-aged and elderly population. Patients may be asymptomatic or present with acute onset of pain in the involved joints (pseudogout, 10% to 20%).[33] The disorder may be inherited, idiopathic, or associated with a long list of disorders (hyperparathyroidism, hemachromatosis, hemasiderosis, gout, amyloidosis, and degenerative arthritis).[6] Deposition of CPPD crystals in fibrous or hyaline cartilage is chondrocalcinosis. Diagnosis of CPPD can be established when two or more skeletal regions are involved. The most common sites are the knees, pubic symphysis, and wrist, though any joint may be involved.[6]

Radiographic features (Table 6-8) may resemble osteoarthritis with chondrocalcinosis (Fig. 6-13). Cystic changes in subchondral bone is a more prominent feature in CPPD than in osteoarthritis.[6] The wrist is involved in

TABLE 6-8. CALCIUM PYROPHOSPHATE DIHYDRATE DEPOSITION DISEASE: RADIOGRAPHIC FEATURES[6,33]

Normal bone density
Joint space narrowing
Chondrocalcinosis
Subchondral cysts
Bilateral involvement
Distribution: Knees and pubic symphysis. MCP joints (2nd and 3rd most common), triangular fibrocartilage and cartilage of lunate and triquetrum.

MCP, metacarpophalangeal.

TABLE 6-9. HEMACHROMATOSIS: RADIOGRAPHIC FEATURES[6,33]

Normal bone mineral
Joint space narrowing
Subchondral cysts
Chondrocalcinosis
Prominent medial osteophytes
Bilateral asymmetric involvement
Distribution: Hand, wrist, hip, knee 2nd and 3rd MCP joints predominate.

MCP, metacarpophalangeal.

65% of patients. MCP involvement also occurs, most commonly in the second and third MCP joints.[6,33] However, the fourth and fifth MCP joints are more often involved in CPPD than in hemachromatosis.[33]

HEMACHROMATOSIS

Hemachromatosis is an inherited disorder resulting in iron deposition in multiple organs throughout the body. Joint involvement is reported in up to 50% of patients. Joint disease resembles osteoarthritis with chondrocalcinosis frequently associated. Like CPPD, subchondral cysts are common (Table 6-9).[33]

Radiographic changes are common in the hand and wrist, and may assist in the proper diagnosis or differentiation from CPPD and osteoarthritis. There is a defined predilection for involvement of the second and third MCP joints with medial osteophytes (Fig. 6-14). The interphalangeal joints are typically not involved, unlike osteoarthritis.[6]

PIGMENTED VILLONODULAR SYNOVITIS

Pigmented villonodular synovitis (PVNS) is a monoarticular synovial proliferative disorder that typically affects large joints in adults (30 to 50 years of age). The knee is most commonly affected. Patients present with swelling

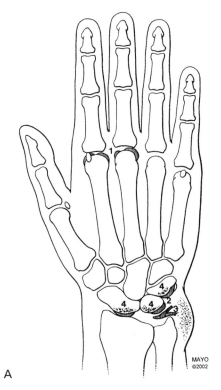

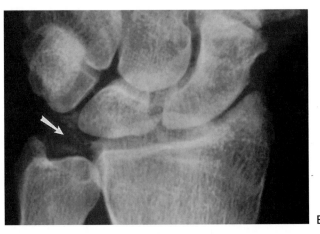

FIGURE 6-13. Calcium pyrophosphate deposition disease (CPPD). **A:** Illustration of changes with calcification in the articular cartilage of the second and third metacarpal heads (1), the proximal carpal bones, especially the lunate and triquetrum (2), the triangular fibrocartilage (TFC) (3), and multiple small cysts (4). **B:** Radiograph of the wrist demonstrating calcifications in the TFC and lunotriquetral ligament region *(arrow)*.

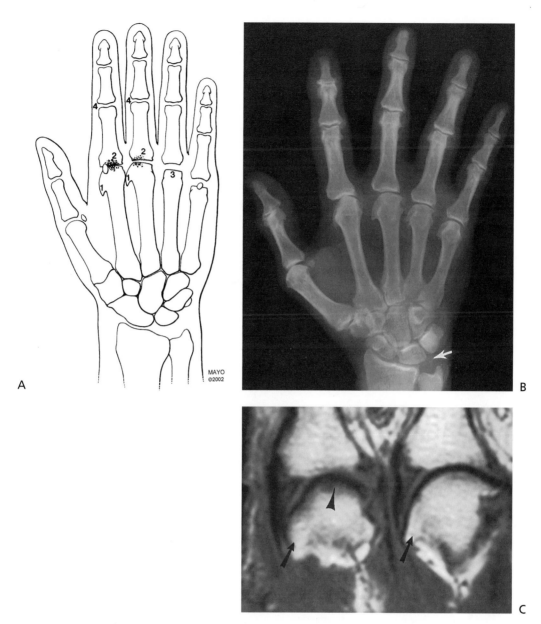

FIGURE 6-14. Hemachromatosis. **A:** Illustration of radiographic changes with prominent osteo-phytes on the second and third metacarpal heads (1), multiple small cysts (20, flattening of the metacarpal heads (3), and sparing of the interphalangeal joints (4). **B:** Posteroanterior radiograph demonstrates prominent osteophytes and MCP joint narrowing with relative sparing of the inter-phalangeal joints. There is faint chondrocalcinosis in the wrist *(arrow)*. **C:** Coronal T1-weighted MR image demonstrates narrowed second and third MCP joints with prominent osteophytes *(arrows)* and subchondral sclerosis *(arrowhead)*.

TABLE 6-10. PIGMENTED VILLONODULAR SYNOVITIS: RADIOGRAPHIC FEATURES[6,33]

Normal bone density
Swelling and joint effusion
Prominent erosions
Cystic changes
Monoarticular
Distribution: Predilection for large joints and lower extremity.

and pain in the involved joint.[33] Joint fluid is characteristically brown due to chronic hemorrhage. Synovial histology is similar to that of giant cell tumors of the tendon sheath.

Radiographic features (Table 6-10) include swelling with joint effusion. Density of the fluid may appear increased due to chronic hemorrhage. Bone density is usually normal. Prominent bone erosions or cysts are not uncommon.[33] MRI features are often characteristic in this condition. These findings will be discussed later as we address the role of MRI for evaluation of arthropathies.

MULTICENTRIC RETICULOHISTIOCYTOSIS

Multicentric reticulohistiocytosis is a condition of unknown etiology that affects adults. The disorder is characterized by histiocytic proliferation involving the skin, subcutaneous tissues, mucosa, synovium, and even bone. Arthropathy may be the initial presenting complaint. Women are more commonly involved than men.[33]

Radiographic changes are most common in the phalangeal joints of the hand (Table 6-11). The wrists and lower extremities may also be involved. Distribution is typically bilateral and symmetric, similar to rheumatoid arthritis. However, joint involvement is more aggressive and distal phalangeal involvement more common than in rheumatoid arthritis. There is no new bone formation in multicentric reticulohistiocytosis, which is useful in distinguishing this condition from spondyloarthropathies discussed earlier. Ankylosis does not occur.[33]

TABLE 6-11. MULTICENTRIC ROTICULO HISTIOCYTOSIS RADIOGRAPHIC FEATURES[33]

Normal bone density
No bone proliferation or ankylosis
Aggressive erosive changes
Joint space narrowed or widened
Bilateral symmetric involvement
Distribution: Upper extremity more commonly involved. Phalangeal joints of the hand with DIP involvement.

DIP, distal interphalangeal.

CONNECTIVE TISSUE DISEASES

There are multiple connective tissue diseases (Fig. 6-15) that may affect the hand and wrist (Table 6-1).[6,24,33] These conditions affect multiple organ systems, and joint and soft-tissue involvement is common.

Patients with systemic lupus erythematosus (SLE) have joint involvement in up to 90% of cases.[6] These patients typically have subluxations without articular erosions, unlike patients with rheumatoid arthritis (Fig. 6-15B, C). Patients with SLE may also have osteonecrosis and soft-tissue calcifications. Osteopenia is also a common radiographic feature.[6,33]

Nearly 50% of patients with scleroderma have articular symptoms. Though patients may have interphalangeal joint erosions, changes in the tufts and soft tissues are most characteristic (Fig. 6-15D). Up to 80% of patients have erosion of the tuft of the distal phalanx and soft-tissue atrophy. Soft-tissue calcifications in this region are also characteristic.[6] Soft-tissue calcifications may be seen as areas of low signal intensity on MR images.[5]

Patients with dermatomyositis may demonstrate soft-tissue calcifications. These are typically along fascial planes, but may also be subcutaneous or about joints. Dermatomyositis involves the skin and muscle while polymyositis involves only the muscle.[33] Patients with typical polymyositis are usually female (F/M = 2:1) in their thirties or forties who present with muscle weakness. Typical dermatomyositis is also more common in females. Patients present with muscle weakness and a diffuse erythematous skin rash. Dermatomyositis with malignancy is more common in males older than 40 years. Up to 25% of patients develop malignancy. Dermatomyositis and polymyositis may also occur in children and adolescents (20% of cases). Again, these disorders are more common in females.[33]

Patients with mixed connective tissue disease present with features of rheumatoid arthritis, scleroderma, and SLE.[6]

POSTOPERATIVE ARTHROPATHY

Following surgical procedures, specifically silicone implants, additional inflammatory arthropathies may become evident.[2,7,8,41] Potential complications include implant failure, infection (see Chapter 7), silicone synovitis, and silicone adenopathy.[8]

Silicone synovitis is related to shedding of silicone particles and can occur in any operative site. However, the condition is most common following scaphoid (75%), lunate (55%), and scapholunate (75%) implants. Patients present with pain and swelling, which typically occurs 6 to 9 months following the joint replacement procedure.[7,8] Radiographs demonstrate fragmentation of the prosthesis, swelling, and osteolysis.[8]

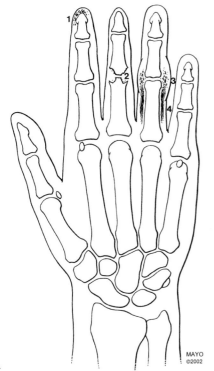

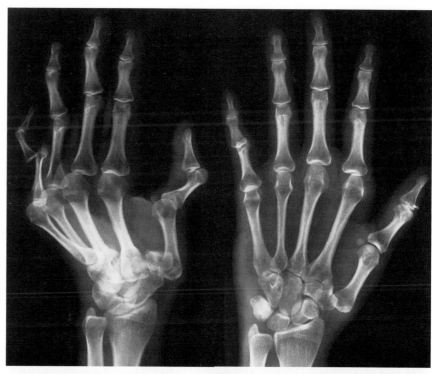

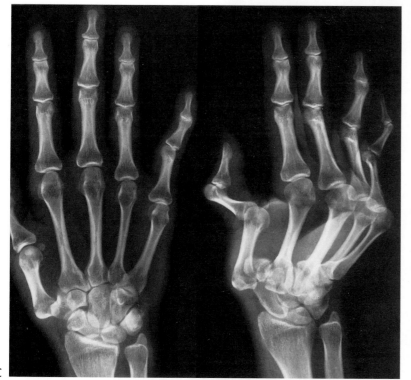

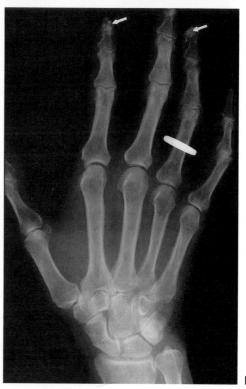

FIGURE 6-15. Connective tissue diseases. **A:** Illustration of common radiographic features seen with connective tissue diseases. Tissue atrophy and tuft calcifications associated with scleroderma (1), joint erosions (2), periarticular calcifications (3), and calcifications along tissue planes (4). **B, C:** Systemic lupus erythematosus. Radiographs of the left **(B)** and right **(C)** hands and wrists demonstrate multiple subluxations without erosions. **D:** Scleroderma. Radiograph of the hand shows calcifications in the finger tips *(arrows)* with soft-tissue atrophy.

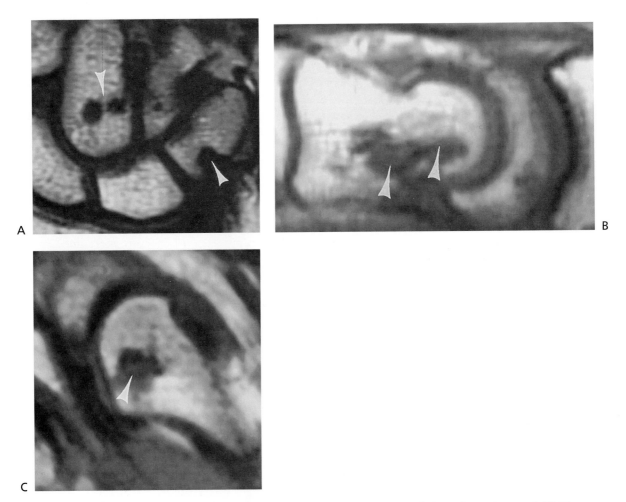

FIGURE 6-16. Coronal **(A)** and sagittal **(B)** T1-weighted images of the wrist and coronal **(C)** T1-weighted image of the metacarpal head demonstrate early erosions *(arrowheads)* in rheumatoid arthritis not evident on radiographs.

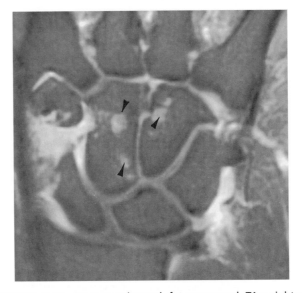

FIGURE 6-17. Contrast-enhanced fat-suppressed T1-weighted image demonstrates early erosions *(arrowheads)* and synovial inflammation in a patient with rheumatoid arthritis.

MRI IN ARTHROPATHIES

The role of MRI in the evaluation of joint disorders in the hand and wrist continues to evolve.[1,5] MRI is capable of detecting bone, cartilage, and soft-tissue changes, including synovial inflammation, earlier than radiographs.[1,11,13,21] Early studies also indicate that MRI may be useful for evaluating treatment, especially in patients with rheumatoid arthritis.[1,13,15,17,43]

Both conventional and contrast-enhanced MRI studies can be performed.[1,5,11–14,16,20,22,44] With either approach, a closely coupled coil, and small (≤ 8 cm) field of view are essential to provide the needed image quality.[5,14,16] Conventional T1-weighted sequences provide excellent anatomic detail and can demonstrate early bone erosions (Fig. 6-16). T2-weighted sequences demonstrate joint effusions and soft tissue inflammation due to increased signal intensity of these features.[3,5] Some institutions also use fat-suppressed T2-weighted or short TI inversion recovery (STIR) sequences for screening of patients with arthropathies.[16] Imaging of subtle changes in articular cartilage may be best accomplished with three-dimensional fast spoiled-gradient-recalled echo (SPGR) or dual-echo steady state (DESS) images. T2-weighted fast spin echo images are also useful for detecting cartilage abnormalities.[11,16]

Contrast-enhanced studies (Fig. 6-17) may be accomplished using intravenous (conventional or bolus dynamic studies) or intra-articular gadolinium.[1,12,14,15,17,44] Intravenous approaches are most often used for patients with known or clinically suspected arthropathies. Synovial inflammation as well as early bone and articular changes are more accurately depicted than with conventional MRI studies.[1,9,14,22] Conventional contrast-enhanced MRI is performed following precontrast T1- and T2-weighted imaging. Patients are given 0.1 to 0.2 mL/kg of gadolinium intravenously. Fat-suppressed T1-weighted and three-dimensional SPGR (102/64, 60° FA) are obtained following the injection. Using the bolus dynamic technique, the SPGR sequence is obtained prior to injection and then every 30 seconds after injection to measure synovial enhancement ratios.[15,17]

MRI IN RHEUMATOID ARTHRITIS

To date, MRI has been most commonly employed to evaluate early changes, treatment response, and disease activity in patients with rheumatoid arthritis.[1,9,10,12–17,20,22,26,30,39–43] MRI is more sensitive than clinical evaluation for detection of early synovial inflammation.[13] Early detection of rheumatoid changes is important to optimize therapy.[1,9] Contrast-enhanced MR images demonstrate synovial inflammation, pannus, erosions and marrow edema before radiographic changes become evident

(Figs. 6-16 and 6-17).[1] McQueen et al.[20] demonstrated erosions in 45% of patients with rheumatoid arthritis of less than 4 months duration. Radiographs demonstrated erosion in only 15%. The capitate (Fig. 6-17) appeared to be involved early with synovial inflammation and the ulnar side of the radiocarpal joint.[20,21] Erosions were evident in 74% of patients by one year on MR images.[21] In addition to typical changes seen on radiographs, extensor tendonitis is common in patients with rheumatoid arthritis (50% to 60%).[1] Therefore, there is an increased incidence of tendon rupture, which can be easily evaluated using MRI. Ultrasound may also be useful for detection of tendon ruptures in the hand and wrist.[1,42]

Magnetic resonance imaging is also useful for evaluating response to therapy, measuring active synovial inflammation and pannus volume, and defining remissions.[9,10,14,15,26,27] The dynamic enhancement technique described above is useful for demonstrating active synovial enhancement and synovial volumes.[9,15,17] Patients with active disease have more rapid synovial enhancement and increased synovial tissue and pannus volumes (Fig. 6-18).[9,14,17,29] Patients in remission show decreased enhancement of synovium, decreased edema, and no new erosions.[17,26] Serial MRI studies in rheumatoid arthritis may prove more useful for evaluating treatment and disease activity than clinical and laboratory data.[10,26,43]

MRI IN PIGMENTED VILLONODULAR SYNOVITIS

Pigmented villonodular synovitis (PVNS) is a relatively uncommon synovial disorder involving hemosiderin deposition in the proliferating synovial tissue.[5,18] The condition may involve joints, bursae, or tendon sheaths. Joint involvement is most common in the knee, followed by hip, ankle, shoulder, and elbow.[19] The wrist is not commonly involved.[5] The MR features are characteristic and present more specific diagnosis of PVNS than other arthropathies. Conventional T1- and T2-weighted sequences are useful for diagnosis and staging (Fig. 6-19). Hemosiderin deposition and fibrosis in proliferating synovial tissue result in areas of low signal intensity on both T1- and T2-weighted images.[5,19] Patients frequently develop recurrence (50%) following synovectomy. Therefore, MRI is also important for follow-up in patients with treated PVNS.[5]

MRI IN GOUT

Clinical evaluation, laboratory data, and after 6 to 8 years, radiographs are generally adequate for diagnosis and management of patients with gout. MRI is not commonly used, although changes appear earlier and the extent of disease is more clearly depicted.[32,36,45] Also, patients with gout have

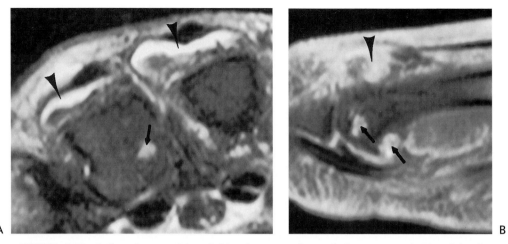

FIGURE 6-18. Active rheumatoid arthritis. Contrast-enhanced fat-suppressed T1-weighted images—**(A)** axial, **(B)** sagittal—demonstrate synovial enhancement *(arrowheads)* and erosions *(small arrows)* in the metacarpophalangeal joints.

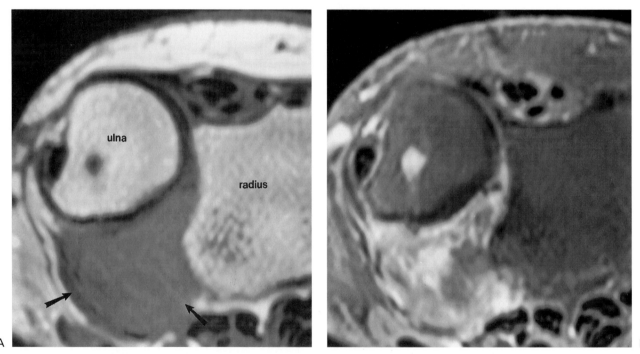

FIGURE 6-19. Pigmented villonodular synovitis. **A:** Axial T1-weighted image demonstrates a muscle intensity mass extending from the distal radioulnar joint *(arrows).* There is associated dorsal subluxation of the ulna with no bone erosion. **B:** Axial contrast-enhanced image demonstrates irregular enhancement.

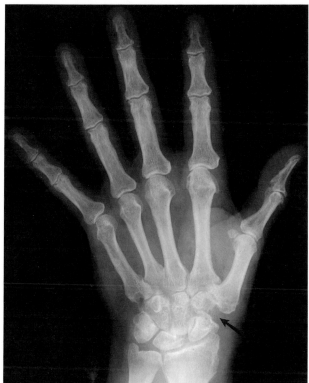
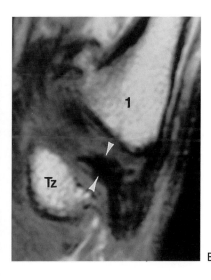

FIGURE 6-20. Resection arthroplasty. **A:** Posteroanterior radiograph shows resection of the trapezium *(arrow)*. **B:** Coronal T1-weighted image demonstrates the soft-tissue interposition *(arrowheads)* between the first metacarpal (1) and trapezoid (Tz).

an increased incidence of avascular necrosis of the capitate and lunate. MRI is the technique of choice for diagnosis and follow-up in patients with avascular necrosis.[5,36]

Magnetic resonance studies on patients with gout should include T1-weighted, T2-weighted, and contrast-enhanced fat-suppressed T1-weighted images. Tophi are typically of intermediate signal intensity on T1-weighted images. On T2-weighted images, the signal intensity may be increased or decreased. The latter is obviously dependent on the extent of calcification and fibrosis in this chronic process. Contrast enhancement of tophi is typically uniform.[37,45]

MRI IN OTHER ARTHROPATHIES AND CONNECTIVE TISSUE DISEASE

The role of MRI in other arthropathies is less clearly defined. Clearly bone and soft-tissue changes can be defined earlier compared with radiographs.[5,23] However, there are few studies of significance compared to rheumatoid arthritis.

MRI has been used to confirm symmetric synovitis in the wrists in patients with polymyalgia rheumatica.[24] Patients with sausage digit associated with psoriasis and seronegative spondyloarthropathies have also been studied.[25,28,31] The primary purpose for MRI in this setting is to evaluate the degree of flexor tendon involvement.[25,31]

MRI is useful to determine the extent of involvement in patients with myositis or periarticular soft-tissue changes in other connective tissue disorders.[5,31]

MRI IN POSTOPERATIVE DISORDERS

As noted above, MRI is useful for the evaluation of patients with joint arthroplasty using silicone implants (Figs. 6-20 to 6-23). These implants have low signal intensity and do not create artifacts seen with metal implants. T1- and T2-weighted sequences provide useful information regarding bone loss and particle fragments in the adjacent soft tissues.[5,8] Contrast enhancement is also useful in defining synovial inflammation and infection (Fig. 6-23).[8]

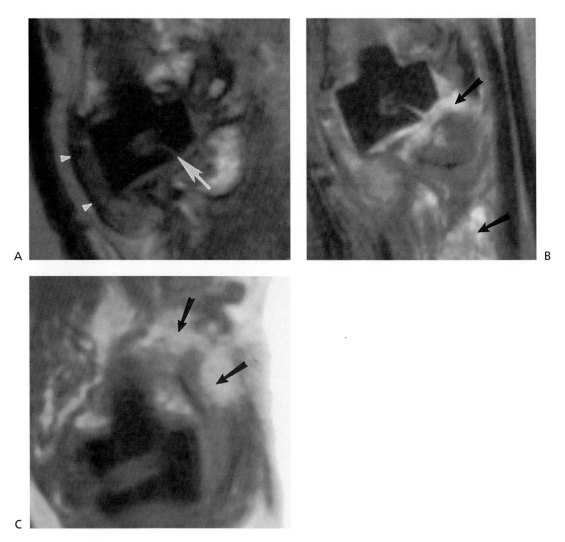

FIGURE 6-21. Single-stem first metacarpal silicone implant with fracture and synovitis. **A:** Coronal T1-weighted image demonstrates the implant fracture *(arrow)* and swelling *(arrowheads).* **B, C:** Contrast-enhanced fat-suppressed T1-weighted images demonstrate synovial enhancement and soft-tissue reaction *(arrows).*

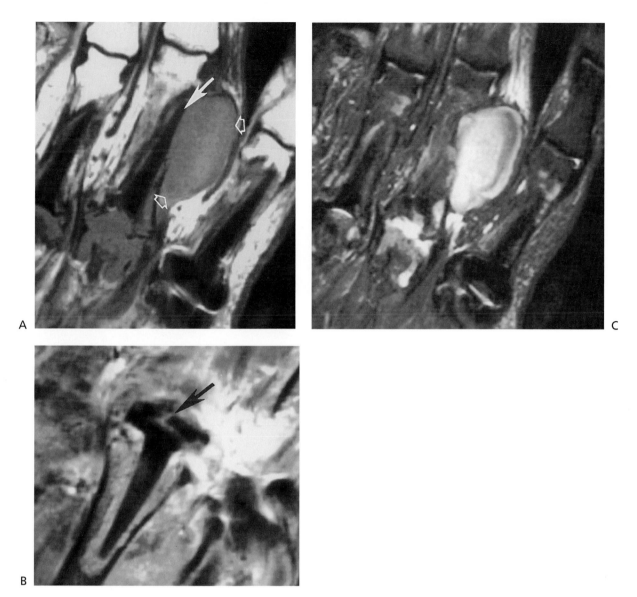

A

B

C

FIGURE 6-22. Rheumatoid arthritis with double-stem silicone metacarpophalangeal implants. Coronal T1-weighted images **(A)** demonstrate cortical break through *(arrow)* in the second finger with a large soft-tissue mass *(open arrows)* due to granuloma formation. Coronal T2-weighted **(B)** and contrast-enhanced T1-weighted fat-suppressed **(C)** images demonstrate fracture of the hinge *(arrow* in **B)** with periarticular inflammation and irregular enhancement of the granuloma.

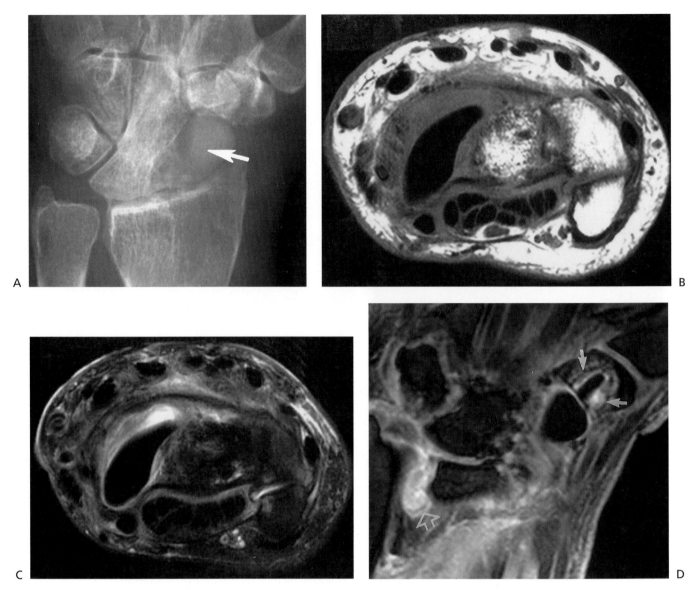

FIGURE 6-23. Silicone synovitis and *Staphylococcus* infection. Posteroanterior radiograph **(A)** shows a silicone scaphoid implant *(arrow)* with lunocapitate fusion. Axial T1- **(B)** and T2-weighted fast spin echo **(C)** images demonstrate fluid around the implant. Note there is no adjacent artifact from the implant. Coronal short TI inversion recovery (STIR) image **(D)** shows increased signal intensity about the stem in the trapezium *(arrows)* and fluid in the distal radioulnar joint *(open arrow)*.

REFERENCES

1. Anderson M, Kaplan PA, Degnan GG. Magnetic resonance imaging of the wrist. Curr Probl Diagn Radiol 1998;Nov/Dec: 191–226.

2. Atkinson RE, Smith RJ. Silicone synovitis following silicone implant arthroplasty. Hand Clin 1986;2:291–299.

3. Beltran J, Noto AM, Herman LJ, et al. Joint effusions. MR imaging. Radiology 1986;158:133–137.

4. Berquist TH. Imaging atlas of orthopedic appliances and prosthesis. New York: Raven Press, 1995:831–921.

5. Berquist TH. MRI of the musculoskeletal system, 4th ed. Philadelphia: Lippincott Williams & Wilkins, 2001:773–841.

6. Brower AC. Arthritis in black and white, 2nd ed. Philadelphia: WB Saunders, 1997.

7. Carter PR, Benton LJ, Dysert PA. Silicone rubber carpal implants: a study of the incidence of late osseous complications. J Hand Surg 1986;11A:639–644.

8. Chan M-K, Chowchuen P, Workman T, et al. Silicone synovitis. MR imaging in 5 patients. Skel Radiol 1998;27:13–17.

9. Cimmino MA, Bountis C, Silvestri E, et al. An appraisal of magnetic resonance imaging of the wrist in rheumatoid arthritis. Semin Arthritis Rheum 2000;30:180–195.

10. DiFranco M, Spadaro A, Mauceri MT, et al. Relationship of rheumatoid factor isotype levels with joint lesions detected by

magnetic resonance imaging in early rheumatoid arthritis. Revue du Rhumatisme 1999;66:251–255.

11. Disler DG, Recht MP, McCauley TR. MR imaging of articular cartilage. Skel Radiol 2000;29:367–377.

12. Gasson J, Gandy SJ, Hutton CW, et al. Magnetic resonance imaging of rheumatoid arthritis in the metacarpophalangeal joints. Skel Radiol 2000;29:324–334.

13. Goupille P, Roulot B, Akoka S, et al. Magnetic resonance imaging: a valuable method for detection of synovial inflammation in rheumatoid arthritis. J Rheumatol 2001;28(1):35–40.

14. Huh Y-M, Suh J-S, Jeong E-K, et al. Role of inflamed synovial volume of the wrist in redefining remission of rheumatoid arthritis with gadolinium-enhanced 3D-SPGR MR imaging. J Magn Reson Imaging 1999;10:202–208.

15. Jevtic V, Watt I, Rozman B, et al. Contrast enhanced Gd-DTPA magnetic resonance imaging in the evaluation of rheumatoid arthritis during a clinical trial with DMARDs. A prospective two-year follow-up study on hand joints in 31 patients. Clin Exp Rheumatol 1997;15:151–156.

16. Klarlund M, Ostergaard M, Gideon P, et al. Wrist and finger joint MR imaging in rheumatoid arthritis. Acta Radiol 1999;40:400–409.

17. Lee J, Lee SK, Suh JS, et al. Magnetic resonance imaging of the wrist in defining remission of rheumatoid arthritis. J Rheumatol 1997;24(7):1303–1308.

18. Llauger L, Palmer J, Roson N, et al. Pigmented villonodular synovitis and giant cell tumors of the tendon sheath: radiologic and pathologic features. AJR 1999;172:1087–1091.

19. Mandellaum BR, Grant AM, Hartzman S, et al. The use of MRI to assist in diagnosis of pigmented villonodular synovitis of the knee joint. Clin Orthop 1988;231:135–139.

20. McQueen FM, Stewart N, Crabbe J, et al. Magnetic resonance imaging of the wrist in early rheumatoid arthritis reveals a high prevalence of erosions at four months after symptom onset. Ann Rheum Dis 1998;57:350–356.

21. McQueen FM, Stewart N, Crabbe J, et al. Magnetic resonance imaging of the wrist in early rheumatoid arthritis reveals progression of erosions despite clinical improvement. Ann Rheum Dis 1999;58:150–153.

22. Nakahara N, Uetani M, Hayoski K, et al. Gadolinium enhanced MR imaging of the wrist in rheumatoid arthritis: value of fat suppression pulse sequences. Skel Radiol 1996;25:639–647.

23. Offidoni A, Celleni A, Valeri G, et al. Subclinical joint involvement in psoriasis: magnetic resonance imaging and x-ray findings. Acta Derm Venereol 1998;78:463–465.

24. Olivieri I, Salvarani C, CantinJ F, et al. Distal extremity swelling with pitting edema in polymyalgia rheumatica: a case study with MRI. Clin Exp Rheum 1997;15(6):710–711.

25. Olivieri I, Barozzi L, Favaro L, et al. Dactylitis in patients with seronegative spondyloarthropathy: assessment by ultrasonography and magnetic resonance imaging. Arthritis Rheum 1996;39(9):1524–1528.

26. Ostergaard M, Hansen M, Stoltenberg M, et al. Magnetic resonance imaging–determined synovial membrane volume as a marker of disease activity and a predictor of progressive joint destruction in wrists of patients with rheumatoid arthritis. Arthritis Rheum 1999;42(5):918–929.

27. Ostergaard M, Hansen M, Stoltenberg M, et al. Quantitive assessment of the synovial membrane in the rheumatoid wrist: an easily obtained MRI score reflects the synovial volume. Br J Rheumatol 1996;35:965–971.

28. Padula A, Salvarani C, Barozzi L, et al. Dactylitis involving the synovial sheaths in the palm of the hand: two more cases studied by magnetic resonance imaging. Ann Rheum Dis 1998;57(1):61–62.

29. Partik B, Rand T, Pretterklieber ML, et al. Patterns of gadopentetate enhanced MR imaging of radiocarpal joints in healthy subjects. AJR 2002;179:193–197.

30. Pierre-Jerome C, Bekkelund SI, Mellgren SI, et al. The rheumatoid wrist: bilateral MR analysis of the distribution of rheumatoid lesions in axial plane in a female population. Clin Rheumatol 1997;16(1):80–86.

31. Pittan E, Passiu G, Matheiu A. Remitting asymmetrical pitting edema in systemic lupus erythematosus: two cases studied with magnetic resonance imaging. Joint, Bone, Spine: Revue du Rheumatism 2000;67(6):544–549.

32. Popp JD, Bidgood WD, Edwards L. Magnetic resonance imaging of tophaceous gout in the hands and wrists. Semin Arthritis Rheum 1996;25(4):282–289.

33. Resnick D. Bone and joint imaging, 2nd ed. Philadelphia: WB Saunders, 1996:12–19, 195–470.

34. Salvarani C, Cantini F, Olivieri I, et al. Distal extremity swelling with pitting edema in psoriatic arthritis. evidence of 2 pathological mechanisms. J Rheumatol 1999;26(8):1831–1834.

35. Senac MO, Beutsch D, Bernstein BH, et al. MR imaging in juvenile rheumatoid arthritis. AJR 1988;158:873–878.

36. Shin AY, Weinstein LP, Bishop AT. Kienböck's disease and gout. J Hand Surg 1999;24B:363–365.

37. Pritzer CE, Dalinka MK, Kressel HY. Magnetic resonance imaging of pigmented villonodular synovitis: a report of two cases. Skel Radiol 1987;16:316–319.

38. Sueyoshi E, Uetani M, Hayashi K, et al. Tuberculous tenosynovitis of the wrist: MRI findings in three patients. Skel Radiol 1996;25:569–572.

39. Sugimoto H, Takeda A, Masuyama J-I, et al. Early-stage rheumatoid arthritis: diagnostic accuracy of MR imaging. Radiology 1996;298:185–192.

40. Sugimoto H, Takeda A, Hyodoh K. Early-stage rheumatoid arthritis: prospective study of the effectiveness of MR imaging for diagnosis. Radiology 2000;210:569–575.

41. Swanson AB. Silicone rubber implants for replacement of arthritic or destroyed joints in the hand. Surg Clin N Am 1968:48:1113–1127.

42. Swen WAA, Jacobs JWG, Hubach PCG, et al. Comparison of sonography and magnetic resonance imaging for diagnosis of partial tears of the finer extensor tendons in rheumatoid arthritis. Rheumatology 2000;39:55–62.

43. Tonolli-Serabian I, Poet JL, Dufour M, et al. Magnetic resonance imaging of the wrist in rheumatoid arthritis: comparison with other inflammatory joint diseases and control subjects. Clin Rheumatol 1996;15:137–142.

44. Vahlenoieck M, Peterfly CG, Wischer T, et al. Indirect MR arthrography: optimization and clinical indications. Radiology 1996;200:249–254.

45. Yu JS, Chung C, Recht M, et al. MR imaging of tophaceous gout. AJR 1997;168:523–527.

46. Yulish BS, Lieberman JM, Newman AJ, et al. Juvenile rheumatoid arthritis: assessment with MR imaging. Radiology 1987;165:149–152.

INFECTION

THOMAS H. BERQUIST

Musculoskeletal infections in the hand and wrist may involve the soft tissues (muscle, subcutaneous, cutaneous, tendon sheaths, fascia, and nail beds), bone, and joints. Infections may be isolated or involve multiple sites. Onset may be acute (pain, swelling, and erythema) or insidious depending on the organism and clinical setting.[4,5,7,27,29] Table 7-1 gives a summary of common terms related to musculoskeletal infections.[6,7,27]

Musculoskeletal infections in the hand and wrist may result from hematogenous spread, spread from a contiguous site, direct implantation (puncture wound or bite), or may occur secondary to previous surgery.[4,6–8,26–31,34] Bone, joint, and soft-tissue infections may all occur via these routes. However, most soft-tissue infections are related to trauma, specifically puncture wounds, and skin disorders.[5,22] Hematogenous spread to the soft tissues of the hand and wrist occurs less frequently.[5,27]

The site of involvement varies with the source of contamination. Patients with trauma, surgery, or spread from a contiguous site will have infection involving the adjacent bone, joint, or soft tissues. In the hand, infection may spread along facial planes, tendon sheaths, or lymphatics.[27]

Hematogenous osteomyelitis may involve different sites depending on the patient's age, clinical condition, and the organisms involved. In infants (0 to 1 year), the metaphyseal vessels may penetrate the growth plate. In children 1 to 16 years of age, the vessels do not penetrate the growth plate. In adults with the growth plate closed, the vessels penetrate to the epiphyses (Fig. 7-1).[2,5,6,27] Therefore, the epiphysis may be involved in infants and adults, which results in the joint space being involved more frequently. In children, the metaphysis is most commonly involved. The joint space is affected less frequently depending on the location of the capsular attachment (proximal or distal to physis).[4,6,27] Certain organisms, such as *Salmonella* and *Mycobacterium tuberculosis* (dactylitis), may be diaphyseal in location.[27]

OSTEOMYELITIS

Diagnosis and treatment of osseous infections can be challenging. Early diagnosis and treatment is essential to avoid irreversible bone and soft-tissue loss.[5] Imaging plays an important role in patient management. The approach and modalities employed vary depending on whether the infection occurs in a nonoperative (hematogenous implantation or spread from a contiguous source) or postoperative setting. In the latter, orthopedic implants may result in suboptimal images with computed tomography (CT) and magnetic resonance imaging (MRI).[4,5]

Routine radiographs should be obtained initially in patients with suspected osteomyelitis. Radiographic changes may be nonspecific in the early stages. Localized soft-tissue swelling and distortion of soft-tissue or fat planes may be the only findings (Fig. 7-2). Bone changes are typically found in the metaphyseal regions of the tubular bones. However, bone destruction is typically not appreciated until 30% to 40% of the involved region is destroyed. This may take 10 to 14 days to be detected on radiographs.[4,6,7] Also, the extent of bone and/or soft-tissue involvement is frequently underestimated on radiographs. The true extent of involvement is important to determine especially if operative intervention is required.[10]

Computed tomography is more specific for defining the extent of bone and soft-tissue involvement. Identification of sequestra and cloacae is also optimally achieved with CT.[4–7,28]

Radioisotope studies provide a sensitive tool for early detection of osteomyelitis. Technetium-99m methylene diphosphonate (MDP)–, gallium-67–, and indium-111–labeled leukocytes and, more recently, technetium-labeled antigranulocyte antibodies, provide sensitive and fairly specific diagnosis for infection.[5,9,25]

Three-phase bone scans are 90% accurate for diagnosis of osteomyelitis in nonoperative, posttraumatic, or otherwise normal bones. However, specificity decreases when other osseous changes are evident. A negative technetium scan excludes osteomyelitis.[7,9,15] In the setting of previous surgery or other bone pathology, labeled leukocytes or granulocyte antibodies are more specific.[25] However, anatomic extent, especially in articular regions, and differentiation of soft tissue from osseous involvement may be less accurate.[4,5,24]

Magnetic resonance imaging is particularly suited to evaluate osteomyelitis due to superior tissue contrast and

TABLE 7-1. MUSCULOSKELETAL INFECTIONS: COMMONLY USED TERMS[6,7,27]

Term/Condition	Definition
Osteomyelitis	Infections involving bone and bone marrow
Infectious osteitis	Infections involving cortical bone, may be associated with osteomyelitis
Infectious periostitis	Infections involving the bone envelope, frequently associated with osteomyelitis and osteitis
Soft-tissue infection	Skin, subcutaneous tissue, bursae, tendon sheaths, ligaments, fascia
Soft-tissue abscess	Localized soft-tissue infection
Myositis	Infection in muscle
Felon	Infection of pulp of distal finger. Distal phalanx may be involved
Paronychia	Subcutaneous abscess of nail fold. Bone rarely involved
Joint space infection	Infection in joint, may be associated with osteomyelitis and soft-tissue infection
Sequestrum	Focus of dead bone separated from viable bone by granulation tissue
Involucrum	Viable bone surrounding a sequestrum
Cloaca	Tract or tunnel in cortical or viable bone
Sinus	Tract from infection to skin surface
Brodies abscess	Sharply defined focus of infection in bone
Garre's sclerosing osteomyelitis	Nonpurulent form of osteomyelitis with bone sclerosis

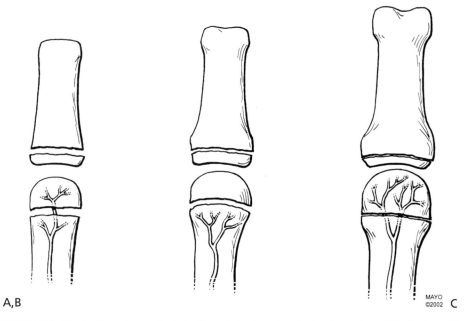

A,B   C

FIGURE 7-1. Illustration of vascularity to the epiphysis and metaphysis in infants **(A)**, children **(B)**, and adults **(C)**.

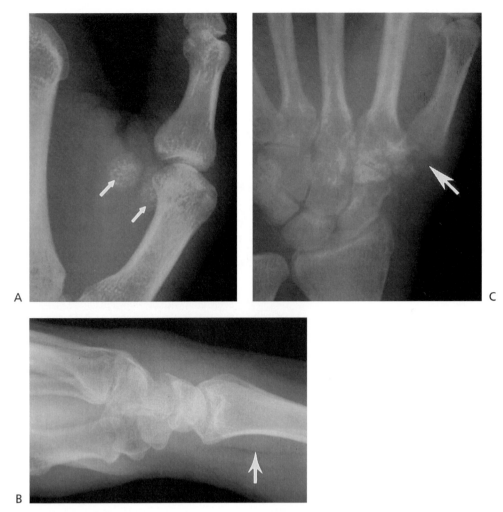

FIGURE 7-2. Radiographs of early **(A, B)** and late **(C)** osteomyelitis. **A:** Radiographs of the thumb demonstrate swelling and sesamoid osteopenia *(arrows)* due to early osteomyelitis. **B:** Lateral radiograph of the wrist in early osteomyelitis demonstrates swelling with a displaced pronator fat stripe *(arrow)*. **C:** Posteroanterior radiographs of the wrist with osteopenia and bone destruction involving the trapezium and 1st metacarpal base *(arrow)*.

multiple image plane capabilities.[5] Anatomic detail is superior to that of radionuclide studies, and subtle bone and soft-tissue changes are more easily appreciated in comparison with CT. As noted earlier, CT may be superior for evaluation of thin cortical bone and sequestra.[2,5,8,12,14,23,31,32]

As with other musculoskeletal pathology, examination of patients with infection requires conventional T1-weighted (SE 500/10–20) and T2-weighted (SE 2000+/20,80) or fast spin echo (FSE) sequences. A small field of view (8 to 12 cm) and two image planes should be obtained. We typically obtain axial and either coronal or sagittal (may require oblique orientation) planes at a minimum.[5] These sequences provide the needed contrast between normal and abnormal tissues to determine the extent of bone and soft-tissue involvement. T1-weighted sequences provide excellent anatomic detail and provide excellent contrast between the high signal intensity fatty marrow and low-intensity areas of infection.[5,7,12,21,23,31] T1-weighted sequences are less effective for evaluation of cortical bone and soft tissues.[5,7,12] T2-weighted sequences demonstrate areas of infection as high signal intensity compared with suppressed signal of marrow fat, low-intensity cortical bone, and muscle density surrounding soft tissues (Fig. 7-3).[5,7,12,24]

Additional sequences may be used or required in certain situations. FSE T2-weighted sequences with fat suppression provide excellent contrast and can be performed more quickly than conventional spin echo sequences. Short TI inversion recovery (STIR) sequences are also useful in this regard, but we do not use this sequence commonly in the hand and wrist.[5,14,15,31] Early studies comparing conventional MRI and radioisotope studies demonstrated both techniques were effective for detection of osseous infection.

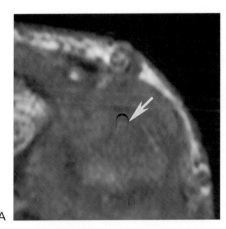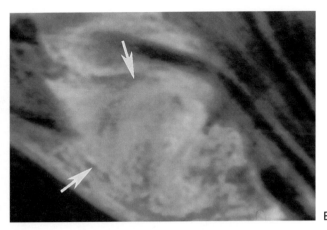

A B

FIGURE 7-3. Osteomyelitis. Axial T1 **(A)** and coronal **(B)** contrast-enhanced fat-suppressed T1-weighted images show low signal intensity **(A)** and enhancement **(B)** *(arrows)* in the first metacarpal due to osteomyelitis with soft tissue involvement.

However, MRI was more sensitive (100% compared to 69% for isotope studies) for distinguishing bone and soft-tissue involvement.[2]

Morrison et al.[24] compared conventional MR, radionuclide, and gadolinium-enhanced fat-suppressed imaging studies in 51 patients with suspected osteomyelitis. Focal enhancement was considered indicative of osteomyelitis. In 73% of patients, the process was complicated by postoperative changes, chronic osteomyelitis, or neurotrophic arthropathy. Despite this, enhanced fat-suppressed T1-weighted MR images demonstrated a sensitivity of 88% and a specificity of 93%, compared with a sensitivity of 79% and a specificity of 53% for conventional nonenhanced MR images. Radionuclide studies (technetium-99m MDP) were 61% sensitive and 33% specific.[24] Most agree that gadolinium-enhanced images are more sensitive and provide improved confidence for detection of bone and soft-tissue changes.[5,18,24] However, other inflammatory or neoplastic changes may create similar abnormalities. Isolation of the offending organism may still require biopsy or aspiration.[4,5] Lack of enhancement with gadolinium effectively excludes infection.[18,24]

Algorithms have been suggested for imaging approaches to osteomyelitis. Routine radiography should be the initial screening method, with radionuclide scans or MRI if the results are negative and the index of suspicion based on clinical findings warrants further imaging (Fig. 7-4).[5–7,21]

JOINT SPACE INFECTION

Infectious arthritis is generally monoarticular in the hand but typically evolves multiple compartments in the wrist.[5,27] Monoarticular involvement in the hand is useful in differentiating infection from other inflammatory arthropathies. As with the small bones in the foot, osteomyelitis and joint involvement are common in the hand and wrist.[5,22] Clini-

cal features may include pain, swelling, and erythema with acute pyogenic infections. Changes may be less impressive with nonpyogenic infections (e.g., tuberculous, fungal).[2]

Mechanisms of infection (direct implantation, hematogenous, spread from local site, or postoperative) are similar to those of osteomyelitis. Therefore, associated soft-tissue infection or osteomyelitis is common.[5,27]

Early detection is essential to prevent cartilage and bone loss with resulting deformity and loss of joint function.[3,5] Routine radiographs typically demonstrate soft-tissue swelling. The joint space may be slightly increased initially due to effusion in the joints of the hand. This is more difficult to appreciate in the wrist. Joint space narrowing and/or bone changes may not be evident for 1 to 2 weeks with pyogenic infections and may not occur for months with tuberculous infections.[5,6,27]

Radionuclide studies with technetium-99m MDP are sensitive but not specific. A normal study excludes infection.[6] Combined technetium-99m MDP and indium-111–labeled white cell studies may be more specific.[9,19]

The role of MRI for evaluating joint space infection is becoming more clearly defined. Early bone, soft-tissue, and joint fluid changes are easily defined (Fig. 7-5).[2,3,5,16,21] Erosions and cartilage loss can also be defined with MRI. However, even with intravenous gadolinium enhancement, the changes may not differentiate infection from other inflammatory arthropathies. Isolated joint involvement may still be the most useful feature.[5–7] The appearance or signal intensity of joint fluid is also of little value. Infected fluid or blood in the joint may have different signal intensity features, but in the small joints of the hand this may be difficult to appreciate. Though transudates usually have longer T1 and T2 relaxation times than joint fluid, we have not found this feature useful.[5]

Graiff et al.[16] evaluated image features in infected joints to determine which, if any, might indicate infection

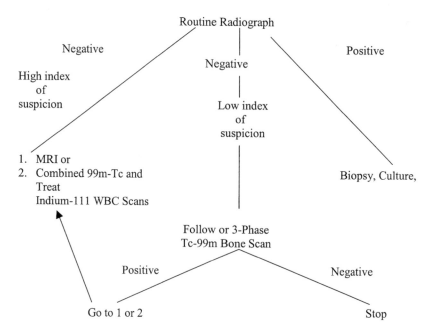

FIGURE 7-4. Algorithm for imaging approaches to osteomyelitis.

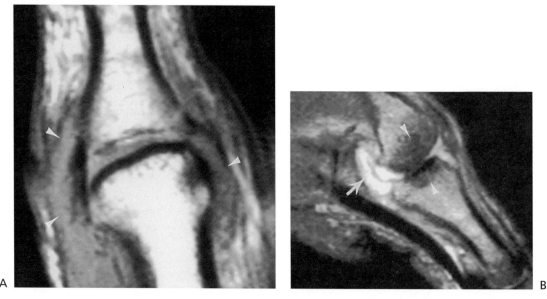

FIGURE 7-5. Joint space infection. **A:** Coronal T1-weighted image shows periarticular swelling *(arrowheads)* with no obvious bone involvement. **B:** Sagittal proton density fast spin echo (FSE) without fat suppression image shows joint fluid *(arrow)* and low intensity in the subchondral bone *(arrowheads)*. Fat suppression should be used with proton density and T2-weighted FSE sequences.[5]

TABLE 7-2. MR IMAGE FEATURES OF INFECTED AND NONINFECTED JOINTS

Image Feature	Infection (%)	Noninfection (%)
Synovial enhancement after gadolinium	94	88
Joint effusion	79	82
Synovial thickening	68	55
Bone erosions	79	38
Marrow edema	74	38

From Graif M, Schweitzer MR, Deely D, et al. The septic versus non-septic inflamed joint: MR characteristics. Skel Radiol 1999; 28:615–620.

(Table 7-2). Features evaluated included joint effusion, signal intensity of fluid, synovial thickening, bone erosions, marrow edema, and synovial enhancement after intravenous gadolinium. The presence of bone erosions and marrow edema were the most useful features supporting infection. Synovial thickening and enhancement were somewhat useful.[16]

Magnetic resonance imaging can detect joint changes early and, when coupled with clinical features, improve the management and outcome of joint space infections. However, features on MRI alone are not specific and do not obviate the need for joint aspiration or synovial biopsy to confirm the diagnosis and isolate the organism.[5,7,12] Figure 7-6 suggests imaging approaches to joint space infections.

SOFT-TISSUE INFECTION

Soft-tissue infections are most often related to trauma, puncture wounds, or surgery. Hematogenous implantation is less common, except with tuberculosis or atypical mycobacte-rial infections.[27] Infections may be deep or superficial.[5,11,33] Cellulitis is an infection of the skin and subcutaneous tissues (Fig. 7-7).[5,11,13,24,30] *Staphylococcus* and *Streptococcus* organisms are most commonly involved. Necrotizing fasciitis is a severe infection involving the fascial planes, but it does not commonly involve the hand and wrist.

Soft-tissue abscesses are well-defined fluid collections that may be deep or superficial. The walls of the abscess may be thick or irregular in comparison with a cyst, and there is usually surrounding soft-tissue edema.[33]

Infections may also involve bursae or tendon sheaths (Fig. 7-8). The latter are particularly common in the hand and wrist.[1,17,20,30] Remember that dissemination of infection in the hand and wrist may occur via tendon sheaths, fascial planes, or lymphatics.[27]

Infectious tenosynovitis may be caused by typical or atypical mycobacteria, as well as by fungal organisms. The tendon sheaths and joints of the hand and wrist are the most common site for atypical mycobacterial infections.[30] The incidence of tuberculosis has increased in recent years due to the increased number of AIDS and immune-compromised patients. Musculoskeletal infections with tuberculoses occur in 1% to 15% of patients with tuberculosis.[1] Up to 50% of these patients do not have chest involvement radiographically, but most have a positive tuberculin test.[1,17] Patients present with indolent swelling of the tendon sheaths. The flexor tendons of the wrist are most commonly involved.[30] Involvement of the flexor tendons may lead to carpal tunnel syndrome.[1,17] When the extensor tendons are involved, the extensor pollicis is most commonly affected.[1]

Imaging of soft-tissue infections may be accomplished with ultrasound, CT, or MRI. Radiographs may demonstrate diffuse or focal soft-tissue swelling. In advanced cases, joint

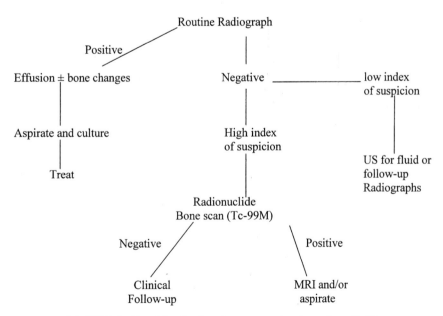

FIGURE 7-6. Algorithm for imaging approaches to septic arthritis.

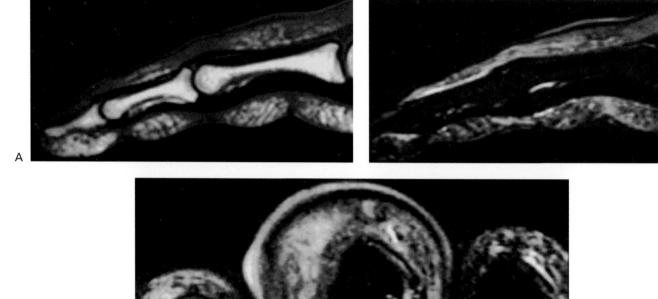

FIGURE 7-7. Cellulitis of the middle finger. T1-weighted **(A)** sagittal image demonstrates swelling and low signal intensity in the subcutaneous tissues replacing the high signal intensity subcutaneous fat. There is normal marrow signal intensity. Sagittal fat-suppressed T2-weighted spin echo image **(B)** demonstrates increased signal intensity in the subcutaneous tissues. There is no fluid in the tendon sheath. Axial fat-suppressed T2-weighted fast spin echo sequence **(C)** shows marked swelling with increased signal intensity in the subcutaneous tissues.

or osseous involvement may also be evident.[5,7,23] Ultrasound is useful for detection of fluid collection, distended tendon sheaths, and aspiration of fluid collections. However, MRI images or in some cases CT scans provide more information on the extent of disease and may have features suggesting the particular organism.[1,17,30]

The superior soft-tissue contrast and anatomic details provided by MRI are ideal for detection of soft-tissue inflammation and abscesses.[5,11,33] Also, differentiation of low-grade infection from other causes of soft-tissue change, such as lipoma, hemangioma, ganglioma, and pigmented villonodular synovitis or giant cell tumor of the tendon sheath, is possible with MRI.[5,17,30]

T1- and T2-weighted sequences may provide the necessary information for diagnosis (Fig. 7-8).[5] Inflammation, tendon sheath or bursae fluid, and fluid in abscesses are high signal intensity on T2-weighted sequences.[5,23,33] Abscess fluid may be inhomogeneous on T2-weighted sequences.[33] We routinely use contrast-enhanced fat-suppressed T1-

weighted images as additional information is frequently provided (Fig. 7-9). The thick enhancing wall of an abscess cavity may be differentiated from the thin wall of a ganglion or cyst. Also, the tendon sheaths are thickened (Fig. 7-10) with tuberculoses, which alone with the presence of low to intermediate signal intensity rice bodies may be diagnostic (Fig. 7-8).[1,17,30] The MR features, though useful, do not obviate the need for fluid aspiration or synovial biopsy to confirm the diagnosis.[5,17,30]

INFECTION IN VIOLATED TISSUE

Detection of musculoskeletal infection can be a difficult challenge in patients with previous fracture or surgical intervention, including joint arthroplasty.[4,5] Radiographs and CT scans may be difficult to interpret in early infection when accompanied by the changes of fracture healing. Subtle changes adjacent to fixation devices (internal or external)

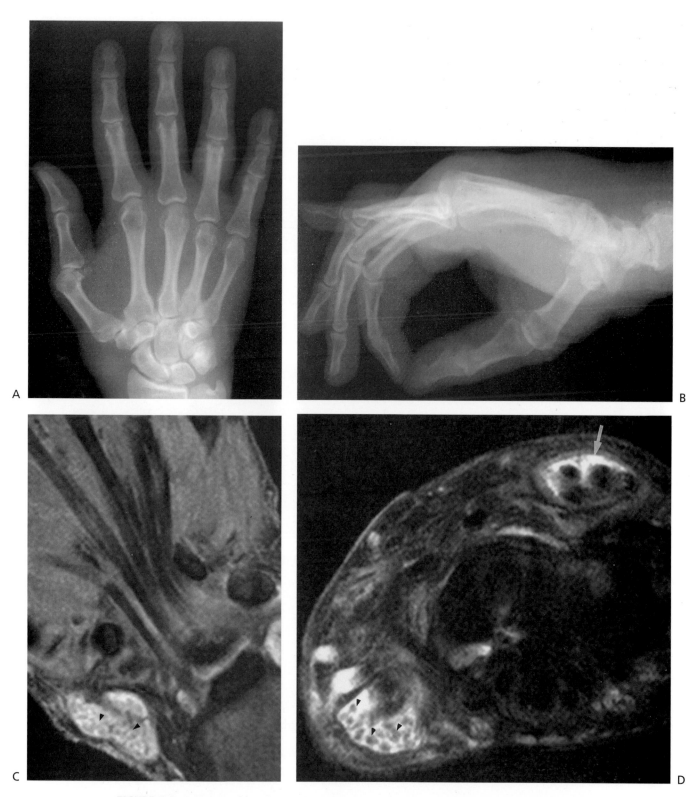

FIGURE 7-8. A 69-year-old patient with *Mycobacterium marinum* infection. posteroanterior **(A)** and lateral **(B)** radiographs demonstrate lobulated swelling of the hand and wrist. Coronal DESS image **(C)** demonstrates fluid collections with multiple low-intensity rice bodies *(arrowheads)*. Axial fat-suppressed T2-weighted fast spin echo image **(D)** shows high signal intensity fluid about the tendon sheaths *(arrow)* with rice bodies *(arrowheads)*. *(Figure continues.)*

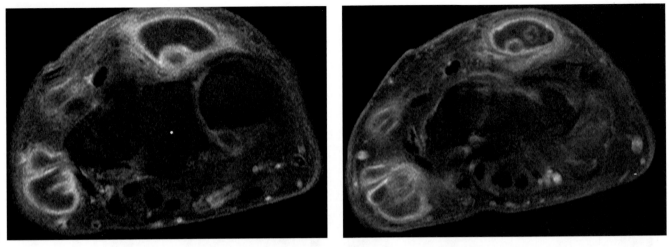

E   F

FIGURE 7-8. *(continued)* Axial contrast-enhanced fat-suppressed T1-weighted images **(E, F)** show synovial enhancement with fluid around the tendons.

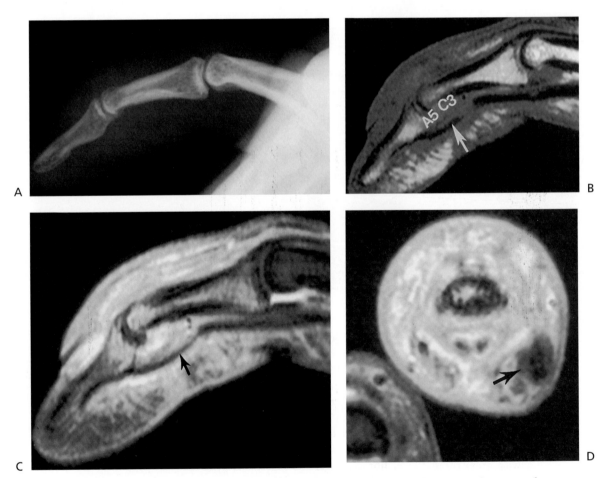

FIGURE 7-9. Soft-tissue infection of the finger with tendon sheath involvement and rupture of the A5 and C3 pulleys. **A:** Routine radiograph demonstrates marked swelling with the finger in flexion. **B:** Sagittal T1-weighted image shows abnormal signal intensity with displacement of the flexor tendon *(arrow)* due to A5 and C3 pulley involvement. **C, D:** Sagittal **(C)** and axial **(D)** contrast-enhanced fat-suppressed T1-weighted images demonstrate the displaced tendon *(arrow)* and soft-tissue enhancement.

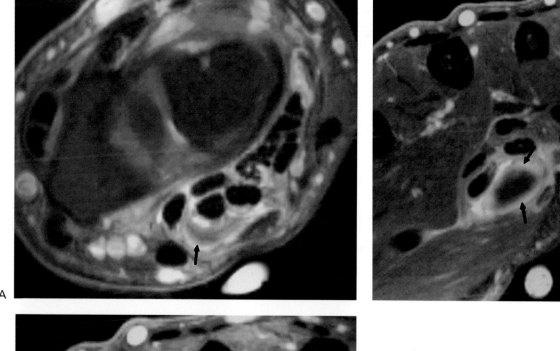

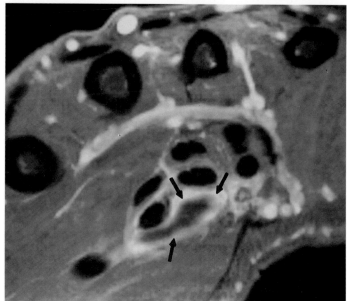

FIGURE 7-10. Atypical mycobacterial infection. Axial contrast enhanced fat suppressed T1-weighted images **(A–C)** demonstrate thickened enhancing synovial tissue *(arrows)* with low signal intensity fluid.

may not be evident for weeks. Technetium-99m MDP bone scans may remain positive for 10 to 12 months after fracture or surgical intervention. Combined techneticum-99m MDP– and indium-111–labeled leukocyte or technetium-99m–labeled granulocyte antibody scans are more effective in this setting.[4,7,9,15,25]

Magnetic resonance imaging is useful for differentiating fracture healing from infection. Fracture healing results in cortical thickening with granulation tissue, fibrocartilage, and new bone formation at the fracture site. These tissue changes are typically intermediate in signal intensity compared with the high signal intensity of infected marrow or fluid. Nonunion results in high signal intensity fluid between the fracture fragments. If infection is suspected, aspiration should be considered.

Gadolinium-enhanced fat-suppressed T1-weighted images are useful in the presence of metal orthopedic devices as artifact is reduced in comparison with gradient echo or T2-weighted sequences. Fluid accumulations such as abscesses will not enhance. However, granulation or reparative tissue enhances to variable degrees depending on the vascularity of the tissue.

Fortunately, many arthroplasty procedures in the hand and wrist use silicone implants (Fig. 7-11). These implants have no signal on MR images and do not cause artifacts in the adjacent tissues. Changes in the joint may include loosening,

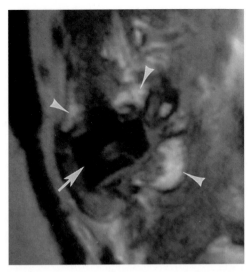

FIGURE 7-11. First carpometacarpal silicone implant. Fat-suppressed contrast-enhanced T1-weighted image shows the single stem implant *(arrow)* with no artifact in the adjacent tissues. There are areas of inflamed enhancing synovial tissue *(arrowheads)*.

infection, or silicone synovitis. The last may be difficult to differentiate from infection.[4,5]

REFERENCES

1. Albornoz MA, Mezgarzedeh M, Neumann CH, et al. Granulomatous tenosynovitis: a rare musculoskeletal manifestation of tuberculosis. Clin Rheumatol 1998;17:166–169.
2. Beltran J, McGhee RB, Shaffer PP, et al. Experimental infections of the musculoskeletal system: evaluation with MR imaging and Tc-99m MDP and Ga-67 scintigraphy. Radiology 1988;167:167–172.
3. Beltran J, Noto AM, Herman LJ, et al. Joint effusions MR imaging. Radiology 1986;158:133–137.
4. Berquist TH. Atlas of orthopedic appliances and prostheses. New York: Raven Press, 1995:831–921.
5. Berquist TH. MRI of the musculoskeletal system, 4th ed. Philadelphia: Lippincott Williams & Wilkins, 2001:773–841, 956–978.
6. Bonakdapour A, Gaines VD. The radiology of osteomyelitis. Orthop Clin N Am 1983;14:21–37.
7. Boutin RD, Joachim B, Sartoris DJ, et al. Update of imaging of orthopedic infections. Orthop Clin N Am 1998;29:41–66.
8. Chandnani VP, Beltran J, Morris CS, et al. Acute experimental osteomyelitis and abscesses: detection with MR imaging vs CT. Radiology 1990;174:223–226.
9. Datz FI, Thorne DA. Effect of chronicity of infection on the sensitivity of the In-111-labeled leukocyte scan. AJR 1986;147:809–812.
10. Demharter J, Bohndorf K, Michl W, et al. Chronic recurrent multifocal osteomyelitis: radiologic and clinical investigations of five cases. Skel Radiol 1997;26:579–588.
11. Du Buf-Vereijken PWG, Van der Ven AJAM, Meis JFMG, et al. Swelling of the hand and forearm by Mycobacterium bovis. Netherlands J Med 1999;54:70–72.
12. Erdman WA, Tomburro F, Joyson HT, et al. Osteomyelitis: characteristics and pitfalls of MR imaging. Radiology 1991;180:533–539.
13. Fleckstein JL, Burns DK, Murphy FK, et al. Differential diagnosis of bacterial myositis in AIDS: evaluation with MR imaging. Radiology 1991;179:653–658.
14. Fletcher BD, Scoles PU, Nelson AD. Osteomyelitis in children: detection by magnetic resonance. Radiology 1984;150:57–60.
15. Gold RH, Hawkins RA, Katz RD. Bacterial osteomyelitis: findings on plain radiography, CT, MR and scintigraphy. AJR 1991;157:365–370.
16. Graif M, Schweitzer MR, Deely D, et al. The septic versus nonseptic inflamed joint. MR characteristics. Skel Radiol 1999;28:616–620.
17. Hoffman KL, Bergman AG, Hoffman DK, et al. Tuberculous tenosynovitis of the flexor tendons of the wrist: MR imaging with pathologic correlation. Skel Radiol 1996;25:186–188.
18. Hopkins KL, Li KCP, Bergman G. Gadolinium-DTPA-enhanced magnetic resonance imaging of musculoskeletal infectious processes. Skel Radiol 1995;24:325–330.
19. Jacobson AF, Harley JD, Lipsky BA, et al. Diagnosis of osteomyelitis in the presence of soft tissue infection and radiographic evidence of osseous abnormalities: value of leukocyte scintography. AJR 1991;157:807–812.
20. Jaovisidha S, Chen C, Ryu KN, et al. Tuberculous tenosynovitis and bursitis: imaging findings in 21 cases. Radiology 1996;201:507–513.
21. Jaramillo D, Treves ST, Kasser JR, et al. Osteomyelitis and septic arthritis in children: appropriate use of imaging to guide treatment. AJR 1995;265:399–403.
22. Lederman HP, Morrison WB, Schweitzer ME. MR analysis of pedal osteomyelitis: distribution, patterns of spread and frequency of associated ulceration and septic arthritis. Radiology 2002;223:747–755.
23. Ma LD, Frassica FJ, Bluemke DA, et al. CT and MR evaluation of musculoskeletal infection. Crit Rev Diagn Imaging 1997;36:535–568.
24. Morrison WB, Schweitzer ME, Bock GW, et al. Diagnosis of osteomyelitis. Utility of fat-suppressed contrast-enhanced MR imaging. Radiology 1993;189:251–257.
25. Palestro CJ, Kipper SL, Weiland FL, et al. Osteomyelitis: diagnosis with 99Tc-labeled antigranulocyte antibodies compared with diagnosis with 111In-labeled leukocytes: initial experience. Radiology 2002;223:758–764.
26. Rahmouni A, Chosidow O, Mathieu D, et al. MR imaging of acute infections cellulitis. Radiology 1999;192:493–496.
27. Resnick D. Bone and joint imaging, 2nd ed. Philadelphia: WB Saunders, 1996:649–673, 684–716.
28. Seltzer SE. Value of computed tomography in planning medical and surgical treatment of chronic osteomyelitis. J Compt Assist Tomogr 1984;8:482–487.
29. Strickland JW. The hand. Philadelphia: Lippincott–Raven Publishers, 1998.
30. Sueyoshi E, Uetani M, Hayashi K, et al. Tuberculous tenosynovitis of the wrist: MRI findings in three patients. Skel Radiol 1996;25:569–572.
31. Tang JS, Gold RH, Bassett LW, et al. Musculoskeletal infection of the extremities: evaluation with MR imaging. Radiology 1988;166:205–209.
32. Unger E, Moldofsky P, Gatenby R, et al. Diagnosis of osteomyelitis by MR imaging. AJR 1988;150:605–610.
33. Wall SD, Fisher MR, Amparo EG, et al. Magnetic resonance imaging in evaluation of abscesses. AJR 1985;144:1217–1221.
34. Watson HK, Weinzweig J. The wrist. Philadelphia: Lippincott Williams & Wilkins, 2001.

8

AVASCULAR NECROSIS

THOMAS H. BERQUIST

There are numerous causes of osteonecrosis (Table 8-1). In the hand and wrist, most patients develop osteonecrosis related to acute or chronic trauma.[2,4,5,8,18,27] Though any osseous structure may be involved, osteonecrosis in the hand and wrist most commonly involves the scaphoid (postfracture), lunate, capitate, and less commonly, the other carpal bones, metacarpal heads, and phalanges.[1,3,22]

SCAPHOID

The vascular supply of the scaphoid places the proximal third to half of the scaphoid at risk for avascular necrosis. The major vascular supply to the distal third of the scaphoid is from the dorsal, distal, and palmar branches of the radial artery.[6] There is a single central vessel to the proximal pole. Intraosseous branches progress primarily distal to proximal.[1,6]

Scaphoid fractures may involve the proximal pole, waist, distal scaphoid and tubercle (Fig. 8.1).[1] Linscheid and Webber[16] reported 80% of scaphoid fractures involve the waist, 10% the proximal pole, and the remainder involve the tuberosity or are osteochondral in nature. Fractures of the waist and proximal pole may result in avascular necrosis in up to 30% of patients.[20] This also results in increased incidence of nonunion.[1,3,16]

Scaphoid fractures may be managed with cast immobilization if undisplaced. Displaced injuries may require internal fixation with a Herbert screw.[1,16]

LUNATE

The vascular supply to the lunate is tenuous resulting in avascular necrosis (Kienböck's disease) relatively commonly in comparison with other osseous structures in the hand and wrist.[6,9,14,15]

The dorsal vascular supply to the lunate is provided by a branch of the radial artery that arises distal to the dorsal artery to the index finger. Branches from the radiocarpal arch and dorsal branch of the interosseous artery may also supply the dorsal lunate.[6,14,15] The palmar vascular supply occurs

from branches of the anterior interosseous artery, recurrent branches of the deep palmar arch, and direct branches from the radial and ulnar arteries. The vascular supply may be predominately from the dorsal or palmar vessels.[6,18,21]

Several vascular patterns have been described specifically as they relate to lunate fractures.[9,14,15,18,25] In 8% of patients, the lunate is supplied by only palmar vessels. A "Y" pattern with two dorsal and a single palmar entry vessel is reported in approximately 59% of patients. Thirty-one percent of patients have an "I" pattern with single dorsal and palmar vessels, and 10% have an "X" pattern with two dorsal and two palmar entry vessels (Fig. 8-2).[18,21,24]

The exact etiology of Kienböck's disease is unclear, but trauma, its fixed position in the wrist, vascular supply, connective tissue diseases, gout, and ulnar minus variance have been implicated.[2,3,6,9,17,18,20,23,25,26] Seventy-five percent of patients have ulnar minus variance greater than 1 mm (Fig. 8-3) and 95% are engaged in manual labor.[3,21] The condition is more common in males than females and typically involves the dominant wrist.[3,20] Most patients are 20 to 40 years of age.[20,21]

Patients with Kienböock's disease present with a history of trauma in most cases, wrist pain related to activity and relieved by rest, and pain and tenderness over the dorsal wrist.[3,21] Patients may have acute or repetitive (occupational) trauma. If one considers the fracture types and vascular patterns (Figs. 8-2 and 8-4), the likelihood that avascular necrosis will occur is more obvious. Five patterns of lunate fractures have been described.[18,25] Type I fractures (Fig. 8-4A) involve

TABLE 8-1. ETIOLOGY OF OSTEONECROSIS[3,5,8,11,21,23]

Trauma
Steroids (exogenous and endogenous)
Renal transplantations
Alcohol
Pancreatitis
Small vessel disease
Dysbaric condition
Hemoglobinopathy
Irradiation
Gout/hyperuricemia

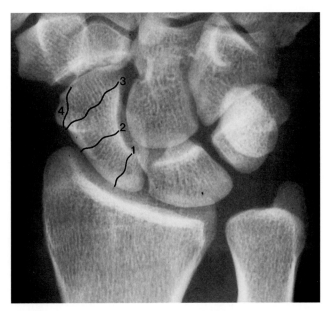

FIGURE 8-1. PA radiograph demonstrating the typical locations of scaphoid fractures. 1, proximal pole (10%); 2, waist (80%); 3, distal; and 4, tuberosity.

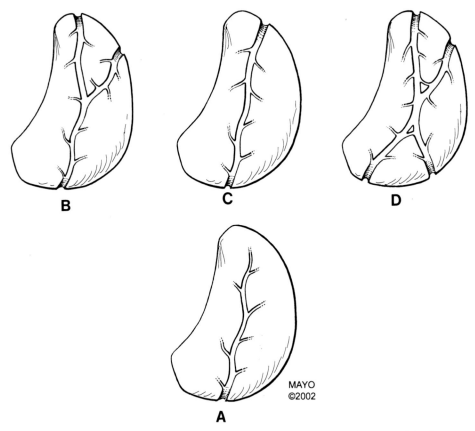

FIGURE 8-2. Illustrations of vascular patterns in the lunate. **A:** Single palmar vessel (8%). **B:** "Y" pattern with two dorsal and single palmar vessels (59%). **C:** "I" pattern with single dorsal and palmar vessels (10%). **D:** "X" pattern (23%)

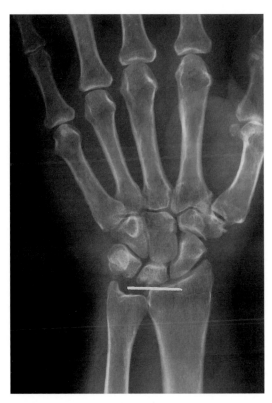

FIGURE 8-3. Posteroanterior radiograph of the left wrist demonstrating 4mm of ulnar minus *(line)* and sclerosis and fragmentation of the lunate due to Kienböck's.

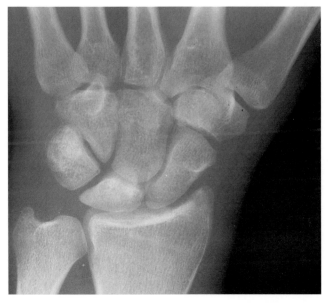

FIGURE 8-5. Posteroanterior radiograph demonstrating Lichtman type II (sclerosis without collapse) avascular necrosis of the lunate.

the palmar proximal lunate and may compromise the palmar nutrient vessel. Type II (Fig. 8-4B) fractures are chip fractures. Type III fractures (Fig. 8-4C) involve the dorsal pole and may compromise the dorsal nutrient vessel. Type IV fractures (Fig. 8-4D) are vertical and type V transverse (Fig. 8-4E).[18,25]

Management of Kienböck's disease may be conservative or surgical depending on the stage of disease and the surgeon's preferences.[3,13–15,22] Staging is based on clinical and imaging features. Though imaging approaches will be discussed in the next section, the radiographic and magnetic resonance imaging (MRI) features used in treatment selection deserve mention. Lichtman[15] described the radiographic staging criteria. Stage I lunates are normal radiographically. With stage II there is sclerosis or increased density without collapse (Fig. 8-5). Stage III demonstrates collapse and fragmentation without (IIIA) (Fig. 8-3) or with (IIIB) fixed scaphoid rotation and scapholunate dissociation. Stage IV disease includes features of stage III with associated radiocarpal and midcarpal arthrosis.[3,15]

Signal intensity changes on MR images are also useful for staging and early detection.[3,5] Signal intensity will be abnormal on MR images even in stage I disease.[2,3,5,24,26] Typically, there is increased signal intensity on T2- and decreased signal intensity on T1-weighted images. The entire lunate or a major portion of the lunate usually is affected (Fig. 8-6).[5] Increased signal intensity on T2-weighted images is seen in

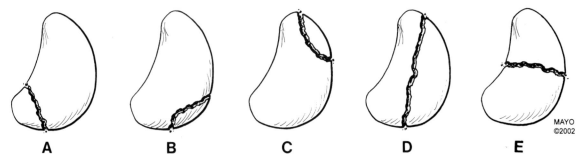

MAYO
©2002

FIGURE 8-4. Illustration of lunate fracture patterns. **A:** Type I—palmar proximal lunate. **B:** Type II—chip fracture. **C:** Type III—dorsal pole fracture. **D:** Type IV—vertical fracture. **E:** Type V—transverse fracture.

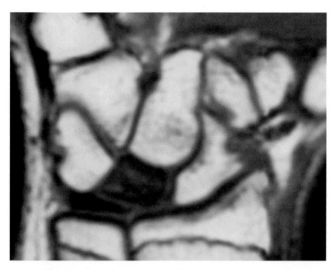

FIGURE 8-6. Coronal T1-weighted image demonstrating low signal intensity involving the entire lunate due to avascular necrosis.

early stages but low or intermediate signal intensity may be evident with stage II–III disease.[3,5,24]

Treatment may be with cast immobilization in early stages. Up to 80% of patients have excellent results after 3 months of immobilization.[18] Patients with more advanced disease may be treated with radial shortening or ulnar lengthening (ulnar minus variance), revascularization, or resection of the lunate with silicone implantation.[13,14,18]

CAPITATE

The vascular supply to the capitate is similar to that of the scaphoid placing the proximal third at risk after fracture.[6–8] The dorsal vascular supply to the capitate is from branches of the dorsal intercarpal arch, dorsal radiocarpal arch, and the dorsal branch of the anterior interosseous artery.[6] Palmar blood supply to the capitate occurs via the recurrent ulnar artery, palmar radiocarpal arch, and deep palmar arch. The dorsal and palmar branches enter the capitate in the middle or distal third. A central vascular channel extends from distal to proximal as the sole vascular supply to the capitate head.[6]

Avascular necrosis of the other carpal bones is rare due to their rich vascular supply.[3,5,6,10,11,22] Osteonecrosis of all carpal bones (Caffey's disease) is rare.[22]

METACARPAL HEADS/PHALANGES

Avascular necrosis of the metacarpal heads and phalanges is unusual.[3,21] Involvement of the metacarpal heads (Mauclaire's disease) may be related to a single vessel to the metacarpal head. In 35% of patients, multiple arterioles supply the metacarpal head.[3,6,28] The etiology may be related to

trauma, steroids, vasculitis, or renal transplant.[27] The third metacarpal head is most often involved (46%).[3,4,27]

Patients with avascular necrosis of the metacarpal head(s) may be asymptomatic or present with pain and limited range of motion. Avascular necrosis of the metatarsal head (Freiberg's disease) may be associated with metacarpal head necrosis.[27] Patients may be treated conservatively or with surgical techniques such as arthroplasty or flexion osteotomy.[5,27]

Avascular necrosis of the phalanges (Thiemann's disease) is rare. The bases of the second and third proximal phalanges are most commonly involved.[22]

IMAGING APPROACHES

Early detection of avascular necrosis is essential to optimize treatment and maintain articular function.[5,21] Routine radiographs or computed radiographic images, radionuclide scans, computed tomography (CT) scans, and MR images all play a role in evaluation and follow-up after treatment. Today MRI is the technique of choice for detection, staging, and follow-up evaluation of avascular necrosis in the hand and wrist.[3,5,20,24]

Routine Radiography

Routine radiographs or computed radiographic images remain a useful screening tool for fracture detection. In addition, radiographic features have been used to stage avascular necrosis, specifically in Kienböck's disease (Figs. 8-3 and 8-5).[5,15,18] After fractures of the scaphoid and capitate, the proximal fragments are at risk for avascular necrosis. Edema in the fragment due to the hyperemia may result in osteopenia. This is a positive prognostic sign for viability. Increased bone density or sclerosis weeks after fracture indicates avascular necrosis (Fig. 8-7). Nonunion, fragmentation, and arthrosis may result, all of which are detectable radiographically.[5,21,22] Nonunion occurs in 20% of scaphoid waist fractures and 36% of fractures involving the proximal pole (Fig. 8-8).[5,16]

Routine radiographs are also useful for evaluating ulnar length. Normally, the ulna should be the same length as the radius at their articular junction (Fig. 8-9). When the ulnar length is increased (ulnar positive variance), one should consider ulnar lunate impaction syndrome, which may cause focal cystic change in the adjacent lunate (Fig. 8-10). This should not be confused with avascular necrosis. The incidence of avascular necrosis is increased in patients with ulnar shortening (ulnar minus variance) greater than 2 mm (Fig. 7-3).[22] The neutral posteroanterior radiograph is used to measure ulnar length.[5,22]

Radiographic features are important to evaluate when interpreting CT scans, radionuclide scans, and MR images to avoid errors in interpretation.[5]

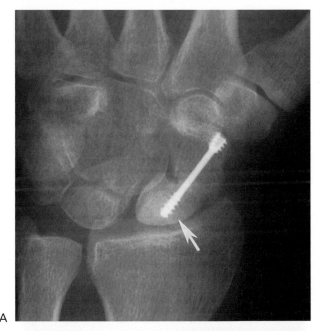

A

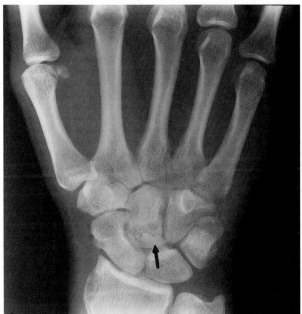

C

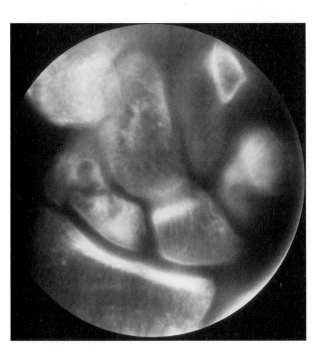

B

FIGURE 8-7. Avascular necrosis after fracture. **A:** Posteroanterior (PA) radiograph demonstrates a scaphoid waist fracture internally fixed with a Herbert screw. The proximal fragment became sclerotic *(arrow)* 12 weeks after fracture. **B:** PA tomogram of an old healed fracture with sclerosis of the proximal scaphoid. **C:** Old proximal capitate fracture with nonunion and sclerosis of the proximal fragment *(arrow).*

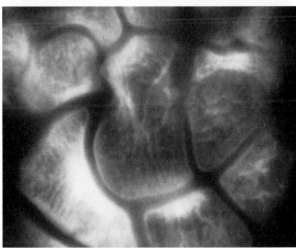

FIGURE 8-8. Posteroanterior tomogram demonstrates nonunion with cystic change along the fracture margins and sclerosis in the proximal pole.

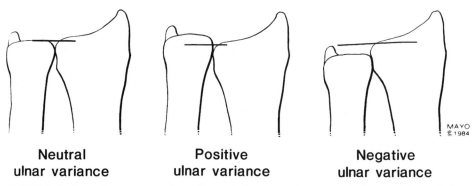

Neutral ulnar variance **Positive ulnar variance** **Negative ulnar variance**

FIGURE 8-9. Neutral posteroanterior radiograph demonstrating neutral, ulnar positive and ulnar negative variance (black lines mark radial articular margins).

Radionuclide Scans/Computed Tomography

Technetium-99m methylene diphosphonate (MDP) bone scans demonstrate abnormal tracer accumulation in patients with avascular necrosis. However, features are not specific and we rarely use bone scans in this setting since MRI has been introduced.[2,5] CT is useful for clearly defining fractures and evaluating suspected nonunion or scaphoid fracture deformities ("hump-back" deformity). CT images should be obtained in two planes or reformatted. This requires thin (1 to 2 mm) sections. Three-dimensional imaging is useful in selected cases. Axial and sagittal images are used for the lunate; coronal and sagittal image planes are used for the capitate and scaphoid, respectively. We do not use CT for the evaluation of avascular necrosis, though others have reported increased accuracy in staging with CT compared with radiography (Fig. 8-11).[22]

Magnetic Resonance Imaging

Magnetic resonance imaging is the technique of choice for detection, staging, and follow-up in patients with avascular necrosis.[5,20,24] Both conventional MRI and contrast-enhanced studies may be used. The MR image features are similar regardless of the osseous structure involved (Fig. 8-12). Normal signal intensity on T1- and T2-weighted images indicates normal vascular flow.[3,5,26] Low signal intensity on T1- and high signal intensity on T2-weighted images can be seen with edema following fracture, transient marrow edema, or avascular necrosis.[2,3,5,26] Low signal intensity on both T1- and T2-weighted sequences indicated avascular necrosis and is typically seen when radiographs show bone sclerosis.[3,5,22] Comparison of MR features with radiographs can reduce errors in interpretation.[5] Avascular necrosis typically involves the entire carpal bone compared with the more focal changes seen with arthrosis or ulnolunate impaction syndrome (Fig. 8-10).[5,26]

Magnetic resonance approaches are similar regardless of the osseous structure, except for image plane selection (Table 8-2). A small field of view (FOV) (8 to 12 cm), 256 × 256 or 256 × 192 matrix, and 2- to 3-mm sections are used. Both T1- and T2-weighted sequences are performed. Conventional spin echo T1- and conventional or fast spin echo (FSE) T2-weighted sequences are

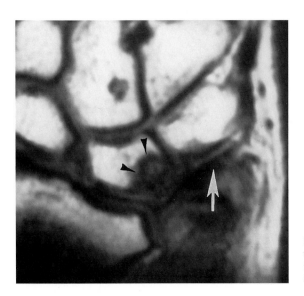

FIGURE 8-10. Ulnar lunate abutment (impaction) syndrome. Coronal T1-weighted image shows distal displacement of the triangular fibrocartilage *(arrow)* due to ulnar positive variance. There is a well-defined low-intensity cystic lesion in the adjacent lunate *(arrowheads)*.

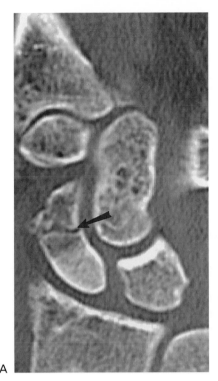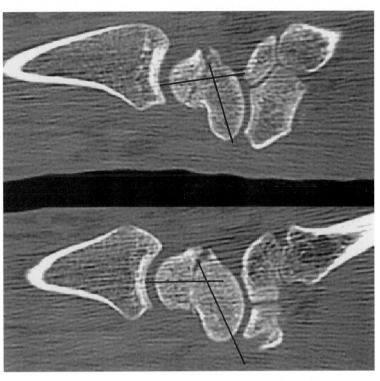

FIGURE 8-11. Scaphoid fracture. **A:** Coronal CT image demonstrates a scaphoid fracture *(arrow).* There is increased density in the proximal fragment due to avascular necrosis. **B:** Sagittal CT images demonstrate "hump back" deformity *(lines).*

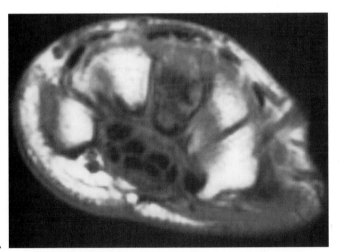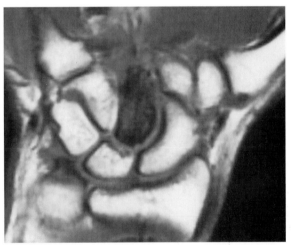

FIGURE 8-12. Capitate avascular necrosis: T1-weighed axial **(A)** and coronal **(B)** images demonstrate low signal intensity involving the majority of the capitate marrow.

TABLE 8-2. AVASCULAR NECROSIS IMAGE PLANES

Structure	Image planes
Scaphoid	Coronal and oblique sagittal
Lunate	Coronal and sagittal
Triquetrum	Coronal and oblique sagittal
Pisiform	Axial and sagittal
Trapezium	Coronal and axial
Trapezoid	Coronal and axial
Capitate	Coronal and sagittal
Hamate	Coronal and axial
Metacarpal head	Coronal and sagittal
Phalanges	Coronal and sagittal

adequate.[3,5] We use fat suppression with FSE techniques. Three-dimensional sequences are usually not necessary. Contrast-enhanced images with fat-suppressed T1-weighted sequences should be performed in both image planes (Table 8-2).[3,5,16,18,19,22]

Scaphoid fractures imaged in the oblique sagittal and coronal planes permit evaluation of fragment position, avascular necrosis, and nonunion.[5,11,19] In the immediate post-fracture period, edema is present about the fracture line seen as low intensity on T1- (Fig. 8-13) and high signal intensity on T2-weighted sequences. Contrast-enhanced MR images are useful in early and follow-up studies.[19] If flow to the proximal fragment is intact, the fragment will enhance. Signal intensity between the fragments is low on T1- and high on T2-weighted sequences in the presence of nonunion (Figs. 8-14 and 8-15). This is due to the presence of fluid between the fragments. There may also be irregularity and cystic changes along the fracture margins.[1,5,16,19] Fibrous union is low intensity on T1- and low to intermediate intensity on T2-weighted sequences.[5]

Lunate

Lunate avascular necrosis (Kienböck's disease) serves as the model for imaging changes in carpal avascular necrosis. Radiographic and MR staging features have been described on conventional and enhanced MR studies.[3,5,12,15,20,22,26] Stage I avascular necrosis presents with normal radiographs and generalized or less commonly focal low signal intensity on T1- and high signal intensity on T2-weighted sequences (Fig. 8-16).[3,15,26] There is inhomogeneous or increased enhancement on post-gadolinium images due to edema and intact perfusion.[22] With stage II disease there is increased bone density in a portion or all of the structure on radiographs. Areas of sclerosis have low signal intensity on both T1- and T2-weighted sequences.[3,26] Contrast enhancement

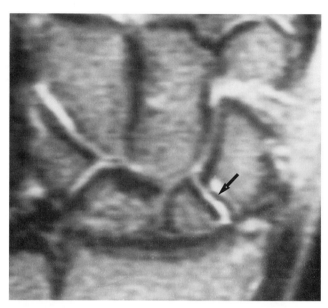

FIGURE 8-14. Coronal T2-weighted image with normal marrow signal intensity but high signal intensity fluid between the fragments due to nonunion.

in this setting is inhomogeneous due to enhancement of only the viable portions of bone.[19,22,26] In cases where osteonecrosis involves the entire carpal bone, there is no enhancement. In stage III avascular necrosis (carpal instability, arthrosis) there is synovial enhancement and irregular enhancement of the carpal bones involved in the degenerative process around the lunate or involved carpal bone (Table 8-3).[19,22]

Similar MR features can be defined with avascular necrosis of the metacarpal heads.[4,27] Unlike the carpal bone changes, early findings in the metacarpal head may be geographic similar to those seen in the femoral head.[5]

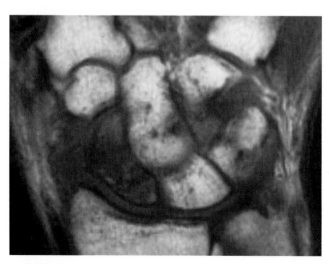

FIGURE 8-13. Acute undisplaced scaphoid fracture with diffuse low signal intensity due to marrow edema.

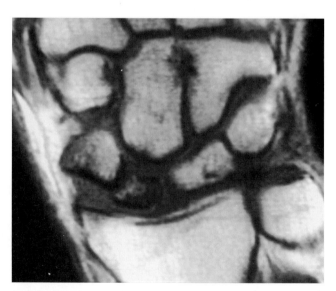

FIGURE 8-15. Coronal T1-weighted image demonstrating an ununited scaphoid fracture with low signal intensity of the proximal fragment due to avascular necrosis.

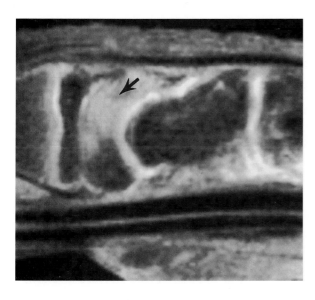

FIGURE 8-16. Sagittal fat-suppressed T2-weighted image demonstrates increased signal intensity in the dorsal lunate due to edema and early avascular necrosis *(arrow)*.

TABLE 8-3. IMAGE FEATURES OF CARPAL AVASCULAR NECROSIS[3,5,15,19,22,24,26]

Stage	Radiographic features	Conventional MRI	Contrast-enhanced MRI
I	Normal	Focal or diffuse ↓T1, ↑T2	Uniform enhancement
II	Sclerosis. Necrotic segment or entire carpal bone. No collapse	↓T1, T2 Sclerotic segment	Inhomogeneous or no enhancement
IIIA	Carpal fragmentation without scapholunate dissociation	Fragmentation ↓T1, ↑T2	Fragmentation; no enhancement of bone; flexion between fragments
IIIB	Carpal fragmentation with scapholunate dissociation	Fragmentation ↓T1, ↑T2 Carpal instability	Fragmentation; no enhancement of bone; flexion between fragments; carpal instability
IV	Stage III and arthrosis	Stage III and cartilage loss, joint space narrowing	Stage III and cartilage loss, joint space narrowing, synovial enhancement

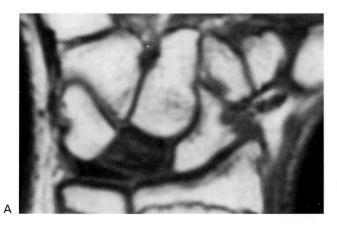

A

FIGURE 8-17. Avascular necrosis with vascularized bone graft. **A:** Initial coronal T1-weighted image shows low signal intensity in the lunate. *(Figure continues.)*

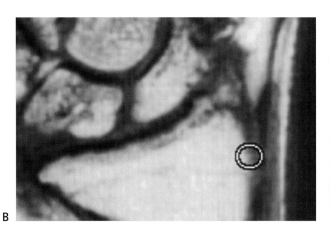

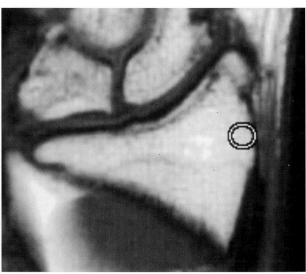

B   C

FIGURE 8-17. *(continued)* **B, C:** One year after vascularized bone graft, the signal intensity has returned to normal.

Conventional and contrast-enhanced MRI studies are also useful to evaluate healing and vascularized grafts (Fig. 8-17). Signal intensity and contrast enhancement return to normal with effective therapy.[5,19]

REFERENCES

1. Amadio PC. Scaphoid fractures. Orthop Clin N Am 1992;23:7–17.
2. Amadio PC, Hanssen AD, Berquist TH. The genesis of Kienböck's disease: evaluation by magnetic resonance imaging. J Hand Surg 1987;12A:1044–1049.
3. Anderson M, Kaplan PA, Dognan GG. Magnetic resonance imaging of the wrist. Curr Probl Diag Radiol 1998; Nov/Dec:191–229.
4. Barnes NA, Howes AJ, Jeffers H, et al. Avascular necrosis of the third metacarpal head. Eur J Radiol 200;3:115–117.
5. Berquist TH. MRI of the musculoskeletal system, 4th ed. Philadelphia: Lippincott Williams & Wilkins, 2001:773–841.
6. Cooney WP. Vascular and neurologic anatomy of the wrist. In: Cooney WP, Linscheid RL, Dobyns JH, eds. The wrist: diagnosis and operative treatment. St. Louis: Mosby, 1998:106–126.
7. Cooney WP. Isolated carpal fractures. In: Cooney WP, Linscheid RL, Dobyns JH, eds. The wrist: diagnosis and operative treatment. St. Louis: Mosby, 1998:474–487.
8. Cristiani G, Cerofolini E, Squarzuna PB, et al. Evaluation of ischemic necrosis of the carpal bones by magnetic resonance imaging. J Hand Surg 1990;15B:249–255.
9. Gelberman RH, Bauman TD, Menon J, et al. The vascularity of the lunate and Kienböck's disease. J Hand Surg 1980;5:272–278.
10. Giunta R, Löwer N, Wilhelm K, et al. Altered patterns of subchondral bone mineralization in Kienböck's disease. J Hand Surg 1997;22B:16–20.
11. Golimbu CN, Firoozina H, Rafii M. Avascular necrosis of the carpal bones. MRI Clin N Am 1995;3:281–303.
12. Imaeda T, Nakamura R, Miura T, et al. Magnetic resonance imaging in Kienböck's disease. J Hand Surg 1992;17B:12–19.
13. Lichtman DM, Mack GR, MacDonald RI, et al. Kienböck's

disease: role of silicone replacement arthroplasty. J Bone Joint Surg 1977;59A:899–908.
14. Lichtman DM, Roure AR. External fixation for treatment of Kienböck's disease. Hand Clin 1993;9:961–967.
15. Lichtman DM, Degnan GG. Staging and its use in the determination of treatment modalities for Kienböck's disease. J Hand Surg 1980;5:272–278.
16. Linscheid RL, Webber ER. Scaphoid fractures and non-union. In: Cooney WP, Linscheid RL, Dobyns JH, eds. The wrist: diagnosis and operative treatment. St. Louis: Mosby, 1998:385–430.
17. Mok CC, Lau CS, Cheng PW, et al. Bilateral Kienböck's disease in SLE. Scand J Rheumatol 1997;26:485–487.
18. Palmer AK, Benoit MY. Lunate fractures: Kienböck's disease. In: Cooney WP, Linscheid RL, Dobyns JH, eds. The wrist: diagnosis and operative treatment. St. Louis: Mosby, 1998:431–473.
19. Perlik PC, Guilford WB. Magnetic resonance imaging to access vascularity of scaphoid non-unions. J Hand Surg 1991;16A:479–484.
20. Pretorius ES, Epstein RE, Daluika WK. MR imaging of the wrist. Radiol Clin N Am 1997;35:145–161.
21. Resnick D. Bone and joint imaging, 2nd ed. Philadelphia: WB Saunders, 1996:951–952, 821–823.
22. Schmitt R, Hainze A, Fellner F, et al. Imaging and staging of avascular necrosis of the hand and wrist. Eur J Radiol 1997;25:92–103.
23. Shin AY, Weinstein LP, Bishop AT. Kienböck's disease and gout. J Hand Surg 1999;24B:363–365.
24. Sowa OT, Halder LE, Patt PG, et al. Application of magnetic resonance imaging to ischemic necrosis of the lunate. J Hand Surg 1989;14:1008–1016.
25. Teisen H, Hjarbock J. Classification of fresh fractures of the lunate. J Hand Surg 1988;13B:458–462.
26. Trumble TE, Irving J. Histologic and magnetic resonance imaging correlation in Kienböck's disease. J Hand Surg 1990;15A:879–884.
27. Wanda M, Toh S, Iwaya D, et al. Flexion osteotomy of the metacarpal neck: a treatment method for avascular necrosis of the head of the third metacarpal. J Bone Joint Surg 2002;84A:274–276.
28. Wright TC, Dell PC. Avascular necrosis and vascular anatomy of the metacarpals. J Hand Surg 1991;61A:540–544.

NERVE COMPRESSION SYNDROMES

THOMAS H. BERQUIST

Nerve compression syndromes may involve any of the nerve branches that supply the hand and wrist. However, the median nerve in the region of the carpal tunnel or the ulnar nerve in Guyon's canal are most often affected.[4–7,13,14,16,30,33,35,38] Clinical evaluation and nerve conduction studies are often diagnostic, especially in carpal tunnel syndrome.[3,5] Imaging is useful to define intrinsic or extrinsic pathology required for appropriate therapy.[8,15,21,22,24,39] Computed tomography (CT) and ultrasonography are useful in certain situations. However, we prefer magnetic resonance imaging (MRI) for evaluation of neural anatomy and pathology in the hand and wrist.[2,5]

ANATOMY

A thorough understanding of the neural anatomy and relationship of the nerves to tendons, vessels, and osseous structures is essential (Fig. 9-1). There are nine nerve branches that supply the wrist arising from the ulnar, radial, median, and anterior and posterior interosseous nerves.[5,10,14,19,47] The nine branches include (a) the posterior interosseous nerve with branches to the dorsal capsule and ligaments. The radial nerve courses along the radial aspect of the wrist adjacent to the radial artery. Superficial branches of the radial nerve (b) supply the dorsal radial aspect of the wrist. Branches of the superficial radial nerve (c) also innervate the thumb and first metacarpal space.[14,47] Dorsal (d) and perforating branches (e) of the ulnar nerve supply the dorsal ulnar aspect of the wrist and anastomose with radial branches to supply the hand. The anterior interosseous nerve (f) lies on the palmar aspect of the wrist on the ulnar side of the median nerve. This nerve sends branches to the volar capsule and ligaments of the wrist. Dorsal and lateral cutaneous branches (g) of the ulnar nerve and the palmar cutaneous branch (h) of the median nerve supply the superficial soft tissues on the palmar side of the wrist. The lateral dorsal and medial cutaneous nerves (i) supply the forearm.[14,47]

The relationships of the major nerves on axial MR images are usually described at the level of the distal radius, pisiform, and hamate hook.[2,5,26]

At the level of the distal radius (Fig. 9-2A), the ulnar vein and artery lie just volar to the triangular fibrocartilage complex. The ulnar nerve lies just medial to the vessels and beneath the flexor carpi ulnaris.[5,47] At the level of the pisiform (Fig. 9-2B), the ulnar nerve lies on the lateral or radial side of the pisiform, passing deep to the volar carpal ligament and then distally into the palm of the hand anterior to the flexor retinaculum but deep to the palmaris brevis muscle. The ulnar nerve typically divides into deep and superficial branches at the level of the pisiform. At the pisiform level, the nerve and ulnar artery and vein lie between the volar carpal ligament and flexor retinaculum in a space known as Guyon's canal.[2,5,47] Guyon's canal begins at the palmar carpal ligament and extends 4 to 5 cm to the fibrous arch of the hypothenar muscles. It is bounded by the volar carpal ligament, transverse carpal ligament, and medially by the pisiform and flexor carpi ulnaris tendon.[14,47,48] At the level of the hamate hook (Fig. 9-2C), the ulnar nerve lies just medial to the tip of the hamate hook adjacent to the abductor digiti minimi muscle.

The median nerve lies deep to the flexor digitorum superficialis through much of the forearm.[47] Just proximal to the wrist, the nerve emerges on the radial side of the superficial flexor and passes forward and medially to lie in front of the flexor tendons in the carpal tunnel.[5,20,47] Size, configuration, and signal intensity in the carpal tunnel may vary. In the proximal carpal tunnel, the median nerve is most often oval. The nerve tends to appear flatter at the level of the pisiform and becomes smaller in the distal carpal tunnel before it divides into five or six branches at the distal margin of the flexor retinaculum (Fig. 9-2).[5,47]

The position of the median nerve in the carpal tunnel may vary anatomically (Fig. 9-3) or with position of the wrist. In the neutral position, the nerve is typically located either anterior to the superficial flexor tendon of the index finger or between this tendon and the flexor pollicis longus tendon. During extension of the wrist, the nerve is most often between the flexor retinaculum and the tendon to the index finger. During wrist flexion, the nerve may flatten and lie superficial to the flexor tendon of the index finger.[59]

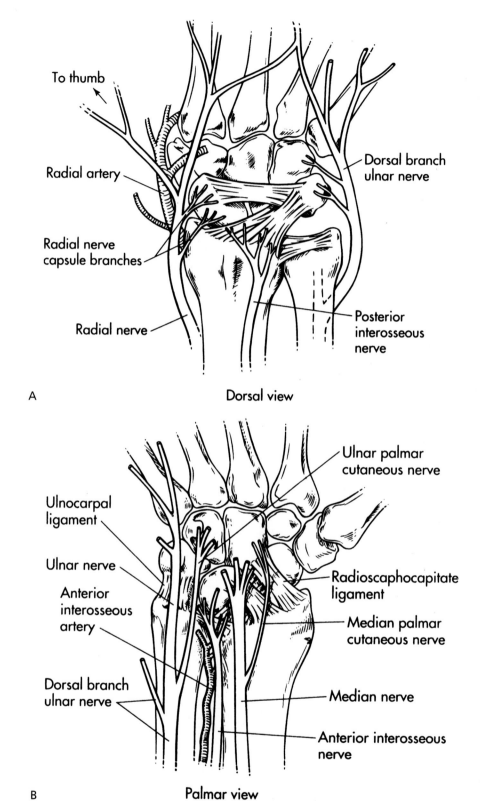

FIGURE 9-1. Dorsal **(A)** and palmar **(B)** illustrations of the nerve supply to the hand and wrist. (From Cooney WP. Vascular and neurological anatomy of the wrist. In: Cooney WP, Linscheid RL, Dobyns JH, eds. The wrist: Diagnosis and operative treatment. St Louis: Mosby, 1998:106–123.)

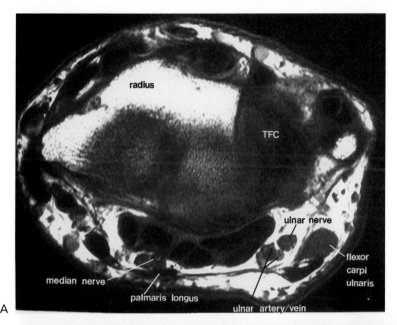

A

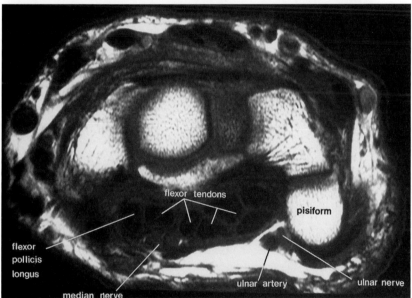

B

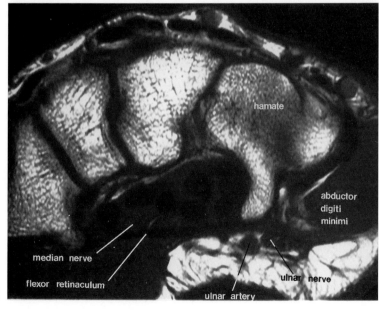

C

FIGURE 9-2. Axial T1-weighted MR images demonstrating the neuroanatomy at the level of the distal radius **(A)**, pisiform **(B)**, and hamate hook **(C)**. TFC, triangular fibrocartilage.

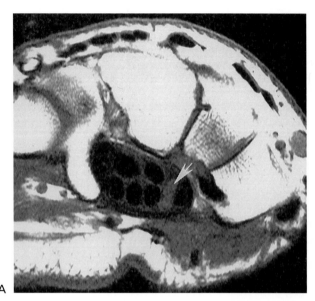
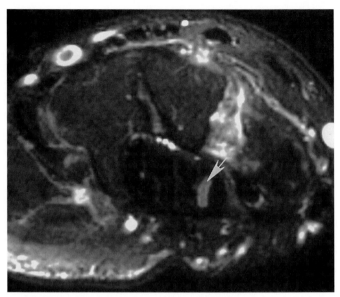

A

B

FIGURE 9-3. Axial T1-weighted **(A)** and T2-weighted **(B)** images demonstrating the median nerve *(arrow)* in a vertically oblong configuration lying between the flexor tendons and the flexor pollicis longus.

Anomalies of the median nerve may occur. Anomalies may affect the accessory branches in the carpal tunnel. A bifid median nerve may also occur.[25,42] A bifid median nerve occurs in about 2% to 8% of the population.[25] This may be accompanied by a persistent median artery.[42]

The radial nerve (Fig. 9-1) descends through the posterior compartment of the arm where it is vulnerable to injury with humeral fractures. The nerve enters the anterior compartment by perforating the lateral intermuscular septum just proximal to the elbow. The radial nerve lies between the brachialis and brachioradialis. Just anterior to the lateral epicondyle, it divides into superficial and deep branches. The superficial branch passes down the anterior forearm just lateral to the radial artery. Proximal to the wrist, the nerve passes posterior to the radius deep to the brachioradialis tendon to supply the dorsum of the hand. Digital branches supply the thumb, middle, and index fingers.[5,14,47] The deep branch of the radial nerve enters the supinator muscle anteriorly and exits the lower margin of the muscle into the posterior compartment of the forearm. The deep branch of the radial nerve primarily supplies muscular branches of the forearm. However, its terminal branch, the posterior interosseous nerve, supplies the wrist and intercarpal joints.[14,47]

NERVE COMPRESSION SYNDROMES

Nerve compression syndromes can have numerous causes, both intrinsic and extrinsic to the involved nerve (Table 9-1). Branches of the radial and interosseous nerves can be affected by adjacent ganglion. Most nerve compression syndromes involve the median nerve in the carpal tunnel and ulnar nerve in Guyon's canal.[2,5,10–13,27,28,35,45]

Carpal Tunnel Syndrome

The carpal tunnel is a cone-shaped space, wider proximally (radiocarpal joint) than distally (metacarpal base level). It is typically about 3.6 cm in length.[40] The carpal tunnel is bordered dorsally by the carpal bones and volarly by the flexor retinaculum (Fig. 9-2).[31] Eight flexor tendons (superficialis and profunda), the flexor pollicis longus tendon, and the median nerve pass through the carpal tunnel.[15] The median nerve may lie volar to the flexor tendons (Fig. 9-2), typically the second tendon, or be positioned between the flexor digitorum superficialis and flexor pollicis longus tendons (Fig. 9-3).[22]

Carpal tunnel syndrome is the most common nerve compression disorder in the upper extremity.[3] Carpal tunnel syndrome in the workplace has increased dramatically since 1980. The cost for compensation and lost work days is estimated at $20,000 to $200,000 per patient.[8] Patients with carpal tunnel syndrome present with chronic discomfort in the hand and wrist that may radiate into the forearm.[3,5,27–31] There are paresthesias and tingling along the median nerve distribution (thumb through the radial side of the ring finger).[27–30] Nocturnal symptoms are common.[5,16] Thenar muscle atrophy may also be evident. Most often, patients

TABLE 9-1. ETIOLOGIES OF NERVE COMPRESSION SYNDROMES[3,5,9,12,16,28,30,45,49,51,53,55,57]

Soft-tissue neoplasms (intrinsic and extrinsic)
Ganglion cysts
Tenosynovitis
Osseous deformities (posttraumatic)
Anomalous muscles and vessels
Ischemia

are 30 to 60 years of age, and women outnumber men 5:1. The condition is bilateral in 50% of patients. Bilateral carpal tunnel syndrome is usually occupational whereas unilateral disease is more often related to space-occupying lesions.[32,54] The condition is typically considered to be related to nerve compression, but ischemia may also result in similar symptoms (Table 9-1).[3,5,9,16,53] Clinical features and nerve conduction studies are usually diagnostic. However, imaging is useful to define the exact cause or when clinical findings and nerve conduction studies are not specific.[2,5,8]

Positive Phalen's and Tinel's signs are useful clinically. A positive Tinel's sign occurs when tingling is noted in the nerve distribution following percussion of the median nerve. Phalen's test is performed by reducing carpal tunnel volume by flexing and extending the wrist for 30 to 60 seconds. When positive, the patient's symptoms are recreated.[5,38]

Imaging of the carpal tunnel has been accomplished with routine radiography, ultrasonography, CT, and MRI. Carpal tunnel views may demonstrate osseous abnormalities or soft-tissue calcifications in the carpal tunnel. Absence of the hamate hook or accessory ossicles have been reported but have not been linked to carpal syndrome.[39] In our experience, the efficacy of carpal tunnel radiography is limited.[5,40] Sonographic techniques have been improved and more often utilized in recent years.[42] However, MRI is our technique of choice when imaging of the carpal tunnel is indicated.[5]

Magnetic resonance approaches to carpal tunnel syndrome may include conventional, dynamic, or motion studies to evaluate nerve position changes and contrast enhancement to evaluate nerve sheath lesions, soft-tissue masses, or nerve ischemia.[2,3,5,8,18,20,34,45,50]

TABLE 9-2. CARPAL TUNNEL SYNDROME FEATURES EVALUATED ON MRI[3,10–13,15,22,24,40,43]

Median nerve shape: flattening, swelling, deformed
Increased signal intensity median nerve
Bowing of flexor retinaculum
Deep palmar bursitis
Tenosynovitis
Soft-tissue masses
Increased muscle signal intensity
Carpal tunnel contents/volume ratios
Carpal tunnel volume/wrist volume ratios

Conventional MRI studies are performed using a small field of view (8 to 12 cm), 3- to 4-mm-thick sections, 256 × 256 or 256 × 192 matrix, and typically one acquisition. Axial T1- and T2- weighted images are best to evaluate the anatomy and screen for pathology in the carpal tunnel. Fast spin echo T2-weighted sequences can be substituted for conventional spin echo sequences.[5,40] Additional image planes and pulse sequences may be needed for perineural lesions. However, the axial plane is best to evaluate the median nerve.[2,5,10–13,24]

Magnetic resonance imaging features in patients with carpal tunnel syndrome may be directly related to the nerve (size, shape, signal intensity) or the contents of the carpal tunnel (Table 9-2). Pathology involving the nerve, such as nerve sheath tumors or fibrolipomatous hamartomas of the median nerve (Fig. 9-4), are usually easily appreciated.[5,7,30,35] Changes in size, shape, and signal intensity may also be seen on axial MR images (Fig. 9-5). The nerve is typically oval in the proximal carpal tunnel, becoming flatter at the pisiform level and smaller in the distal carpal tunnel.[47] Swelling

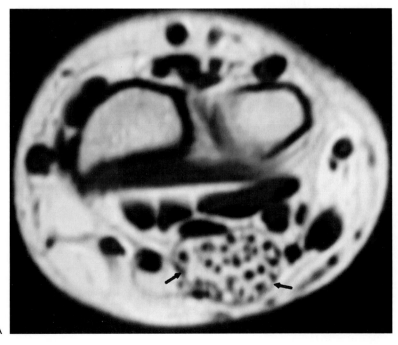

A

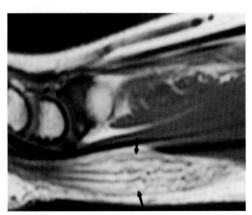

B

FIGURE 9-4. Fibrolipomatous hamartoma of the median nerve. Axial **(A)** and sagittal **(B)** T1-weighted images demonstrate a large *(arrows)* fatty mass expanding the median nerve.

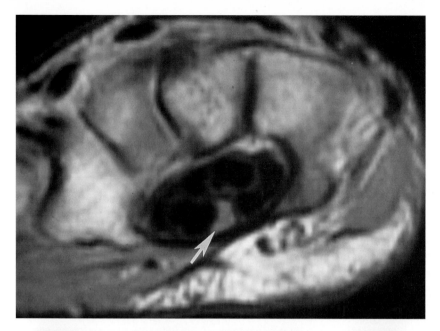

FIGURE 9-5. Axial proton density weighted image shows increased signal intensity and deformity of the median nerve *(arrow)* in a patient with thickened flexor tendons and carpal tunnel syndrome.

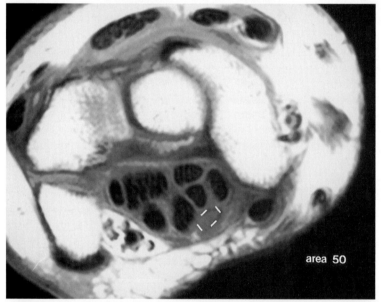

A

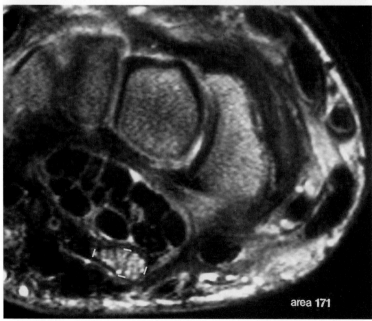

B

FIGURE 9-6. Median nerve swelling, increased signal intensity, and an area 3.42 times normal. **A:** Normal T1-weighted axial with median nerve 10 mm/5 mm *(lines)* with area of 50 mm². **B:** Axial T2-weighted image shows high signal intensity and swelling of the median nerve *(lines)* with an area of 171 mm² which is 3.42 times that of the normal patient **(A)**.

of the nerve is best evaluated at the level of the pisiform (Fig. 9-6). In patients with carpal tunnel syndrome, the nerve is 1.6 to 3.5 times larger at this level than at the distal radioulnar joint.[15,25] Enlargement of the median nerve is reported in 62% to 95% of patients with carpal tunnel syndrome.[56] Flattening of the median nerve is optimally evaluated at the level of the hamate. The ratio of the major axis to the minor axis measurement of the nerve was 1.8 at the level of the distal radius compared with 3.8 at the hamate level in patients with carpal tunnel syndrome. Normal patients have, on average, a 2.9 major to minor axis ratio at the hamate level (Fig. 9-7).[15,29]

Bak et al.[3] correlated nerve conduction studies with median nerve size at three levels (distal radius, pisiform, hamate hook). The width (major axis) and thickness (minor axis) were measured and the area calculated at all three locations. Swelling and flattening ratios were also calculated at all three levels. The flattening ratio is the length of the major axis divided by the minor axis (Fig. 9-7). The swelling ratio is determined by dividing the cross-sectional area at the pisiform level by the area of the nerve at the level of the distal radius.[3] In this study, there was a poor correlation between MR features and nerve conduction findings. In other reports, flattening had a sensitivity of 27% to 65% and a specificity of 70% to 97%.[22,43] Swelling of the median nerve has a 23% sensitivity and 76% specificity.[43] Obvious distortion of the nerve (Fig. 9-5) is usually associated with significant pathology adjacent to the nerve.[1,5,55]

Abnormal signal intensity in the median nerve has also been described in patients with carpal tunnel syndrome.[2,3,5] The median nerve is normally higher in signal intensity than the tendons on T2-weighted sequences.[5,15] Abnormally high signal intensity on T2-weighted images has been reported in 52% to 85% of patients with carpal tunnel syndrome (Fig. 9-8). Signal intensity changes are related to compression and/or ischemia.[5,29,53] Abnormal signal intensity has a sensitivity of 59% to 95% and specificity of 51% to 59% taken as a solitary finding.[22,43] Increased signal intensity in the median nerve has been reported in 52% to 85% of cases.[56] The finding of increased signal intensity in association with swelling, flattening, or distortion of the nerve is more significant (Figs. 9-5 and 9-8).[5]

Bowing of the flexor retinaculum, along with flattening of the nerve and deep palmar bursitis, has been suggested to be the three most useful MR features for diagnosis of carpal tunnel syndrome on MRI.[43] Bowing of the flexor retinaculum is optimally evaluated at the level of the hamate hook (Fig. 9-9).[2,15] The flexor retinaculum is normally straight or concave. Bowing is created by increased pressure or volume in the carpal tunnel.[2,3,15] Evaluation of the bowing is expressed as a ratio (Fig. 9-9). To determine the ratio, a line is drawn from the triquetral tubercle to the tip of the hamate hook (HT). The distance from the line to the flexor retinaculum (palmar displacement, PD) is divided by the length of line TH.[2,3] The normal ratio is 0 to 0.15 (mean 0.10) compared with 0.14 to 0.26 (mean 0.18) in patients with

carpal tunnel syndrome.[2,3,15] The sensitivity of this ratio is 16% to 32% and the specificity 91% to 94%.[22,43] Overall, bowing of the flexor retinaculum is seen in 73% to 85% of patients with carpal tunnel syndrome.[56]

The carpus/tunnel index has also been evaluated to enhance accuracy of diagnosis for carpal tunnel syndrome. This index is derived from the cross-sectional area of the carpal tunnel and the skeletal width of the carpus at the level of the hamate hook. The anteroposterior width of the carpal tunnel (inner aspect of the carpal bones to the inner aspect of the flexor retinaculum) is measured, multiplied by the retinacular length, and divided into the width of the carpus at this level. The index (C/FH × TH) (Fig. 9-10) is 0.18 to 0.39 (mean 0.26) in normal patients and 0.17 to 0.39 (mean 0.24) in patients with carpal tunnel syndrome.[3]

Carpal tunnel contents to carpal tunnel volume ratios have also been utilized to evaluate patients with suspected carpal tunnel syndrome.[10,12,13,20,46] The inner margins of the carpal tunnel are determined at the level of the hamate hook (Fig.9-11).[10,11,13] The individual tendons and median nerve are measured and the cumulative area calculated. The carpal tunnel content to carpal tunnel volume ratios (CTC/CTV) are higher in patients with carpal tunnel syndrome.[10,11,13]

Soft-tissue masses and tenosynovitis (Fig. 9-9B) are easily detected on conventional MR images. Detection of a soft-tissue mass is useful in surgical planning and may be able to predict the nature of the lesion.[5] Tenosynovitis may be due to overuse or inflammatory arthropathies. Infection may also cause inflammation and fluid distortion of tendon sheaths. Findings may be nonspecific except in cases of tuberculosis (typical and atypical) (Fig. 9-12).[1,21,52] Musculoskeletal involvement occurs in 1% to 15% of patients with tuberculosis.[1] Patients present with chronic diffuse swelling of the wrist. On MR images, the tendon sheaths are distended with high signal intensity fluid on T2-weighted images. Rice bodies are seen as foci of low signal intensity in the high-intensity fluid.[21] Table 9-3 lists other causes of chronic tenosynovitis.[1,5,21,52]

Other MRI approaches have also been suggested to evaluate ischemic changes and nerve position changes with motion.[5,7,23,53] When conventional images are normal or equivocal, one should consider motion studies and/or contrast-enhanced images.[5,53,59] Gradient echo images can be obtained with the wrist in neutral and various degrees of flexion and extension to determine nerve position changes or lack of motion with deformity due to adjacent tendons in cases of nerve entrapment.[5,7,23,34] Brahme et al.[7] studied pre- and postexercise imaging using fat-suppressed proton density and T2-weighted axial images. Using this approach, carpal tunnel syndrome was confirmed at surgery in 18 of 21 patients. Sensitivity did not increase but specificity did (87% to 100%) using postexercise MRI.

Most MR protocols are designed to detect compression or entrapment. Ischemia may also cause carpal tunnel syndrome (Table 9-1).[3,53] This could explain why the nerve and surrounding structures may appear normal in

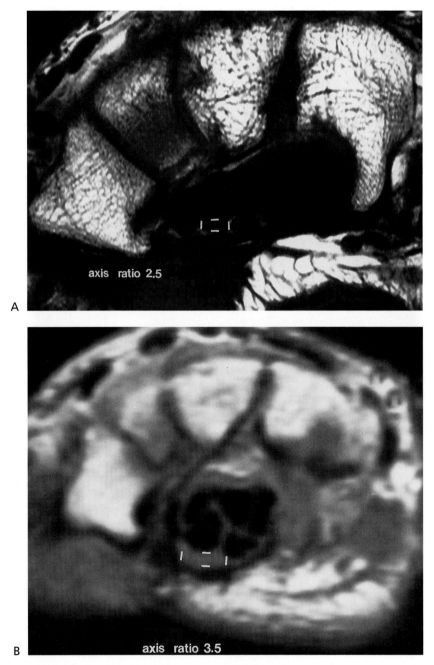

FIGURE 9-7. Flattening of the median nerve at the hamate level. **A:** Axial T1-weighted image with a major (width)/minor (thickness) axis ratio *(lines)* of 2.5. **B:** T1-weighted image demonstrates flattening with a major/minor axis ratio *(lines)* of 3.5.

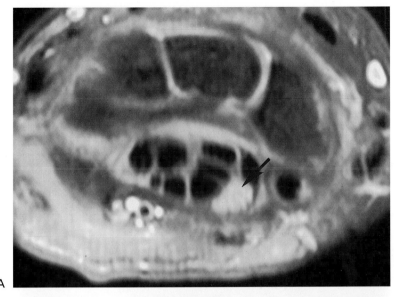

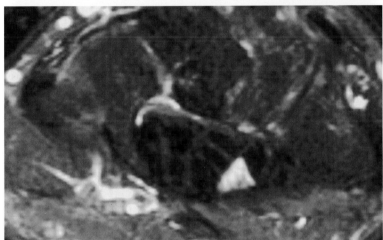

FIGURE 9-8. A 40-year-old woman with carpal tunnel syndrome. Axial fat-suppressed proton density **(A)** at the level of the pisiform and **(B)** T2-weighted image at the hamate hook level demonstrate swelling, deformity, and increased signal intensity in the median nerve *(arrow)*.

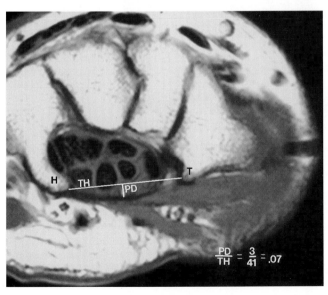

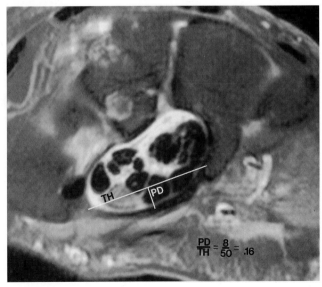

FIGURE 9-9. Bowing ratio. A line from the attachment of the hamate hook (H) to the trapezial tubercle (T) termed HT is measured. A perpendicular line (PD, palmar displacement) is drawn to the flexor retinaculum. PD/HT results in the bowing ratio. Normal 0 to 0.15. **A:** Axial T1-weighted image in a normal patient with TH = 41 mm, PD = 3 mm for a bowing ratio (PD) of 0.07. **B:** Axial postcontrast fat-suppressed T1-weighted image in a patient with tenosynovitis and swelling of the median nerve with TH = 50, PD = 8 for a bowing ratio of 0.16.

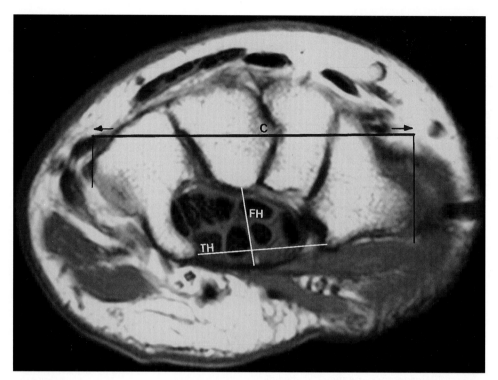

FIGURE 9-10. Carpus/tunnel index. The distance from the carpal bones to flexor retinaculum (FH) is multiplied by the distance from the trapezoid and hamate hook attachments (TH). The carpal width (C) is divided by TH × FH (C/TH × FH) to obtain the carpus/tunnel index. Normal 0.18- to 0.39 (mean 0.26). Patients with carpal tunnel syndrome have a slightly lower index (mean 0.24, range 0.17 to 0.39). T1-weighted axial image at the level of the hamate hook. TH = 41, FH = 20, C = 103. The carpus/tunnel index = 0.13.

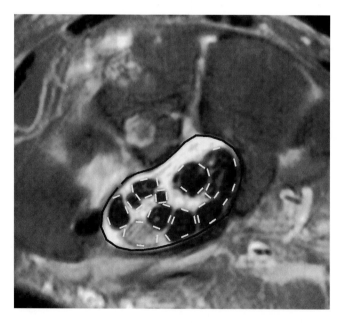

FIGURE 9-11. Carpal tunnel content/carpal tunnel volume ratio. Content (combined area of median nerve and flexor tendons) is measured at the level of the hamate hook (small lines). Carpal tunnel volume is measured using the perimeter of the carpal tunnel (outer line).

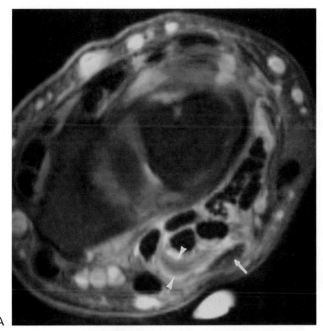
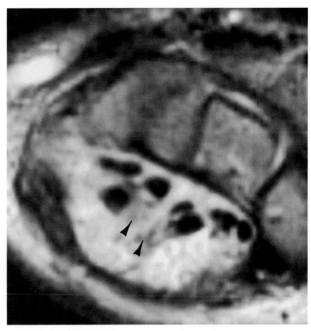

A   B

FIGURE 9-12. Atypical mycobacterial infection with carpal tunnel syndrome. **A:** Axial contrast-enhanced image at the level of the distal radius demonstrates synovial enhancement and fluid *(arrowheads)* surrounding the median nerve *(arrow)*, which shows slight irregular enhancement. **B:** Axial T2-weighted image shows marked distention of the carpal tunnel. The nerve is not clearly seen. Focal areas of low signal near the tendons *(arrowheads)* due to rice bodies.

patients with clinical and electromyographic features of carpal tunnel syndrome. Sugimoto et al.[53] used dynamic gadolinium-enhanced imaging and described two abnormal patterns attributable to ischemia: enhancement due to edema and decreased enhancement due to decreased flow to the nerve.

Physiologic imaging using diffusion-weighted images has revolutionized imaging of the brain. This technique has not been thoroughly investigated in the peripheral nervous system. However, improved sensitivity and specificity may be expected.[22]

Although MR techniques need improvement in terms of their sensitivity, the overall accuracy, when compared with surgical findings, is 91%.[24] When conservative treatment fails, surgical decompression of the carpal tunnel may be required. Obviously, surgery is the initial choice in patients with soft-tissue masses or other intra- or extraneural lesions where surgery is indicated.[5] Surgical decompression can

TABLE 9-3. CHRONIC TENOSYNOVITIS DIFFERENTIAL DIAGNOSIS[1,5,21,52]

Chronic overuse
Rheumatoid arthritis
Fungal infections
Pigmented villonodular synovitis
Sarcoidosis
Gout
Amyloidosis

be accomplished arthroscopically or using open approaches with or without tenosynovectomy.[2,50] In a recent study, tenosynovectomy did not demonstrate additional benefit.[50]

Magnetic resonance imaging is useful postoperatively to confirm complete release of the flexor retinaculum and detect complications or causes of recurrent symptoms. The same approaches used above can be employed. Ideally, the same sequences and techniques used preoperatively should be used postoperatively. A baseline study should be obtained as soon as the patient can tolerate the MRI examination.[5]

Following decompression, MR images demonstrate the flexor retinacular defect with volar displacement of the separated fragments (Fig. 9-13). The flexor tendons are also displaced in a palmar direction and may extend through the flexor retinacular defect. Over time there may be an increase in carpal tunnel fat, and scarring may also occur.[2] This is why baseline examinations are useful for following operative results.[5]

Magnetic resonance imaging can be used to detect early and late complications, including hematomas, hemorrhage, mass reoccurrence, and scarring around the median nerve.[2,5] Incomplete release can be seen as areas of intact flexor retinaculum (Fig. 9-14).[2]

Ulnar Nerve Compression

Ulnar nerve injury or compression may occur in the elbow region, along its course or more commonly in Guyon's canal (Figs. 9-1 and 9-2).[2,41,48] Guyon's canal begins at the

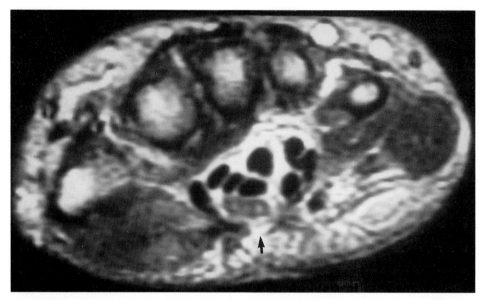

FIGURE 9-13. Carpal tunnel release. Axial proton density image demonstrates the gap *(arrow)* in the flexor retinaculum with palmar displacement of the nerve and tendons.

proximal margin of the palmar (volar) carpal ligament and extends to the fibrous arch of the hypothenar muscles. The canal (Fig. 9-15) is bounded by the volar carpal ligament, the deep transverse carpal ligament, the flexor carpi ulnaris tendon, and the pisiform.[4,48] The canal is divided into three zones, with symptoms related to the zone involved.[40] Zone 1 is the proximal portion of the canal before the bifurcation of the ulnar nerve. Injury or compression in this zone leads to motor and sensory deficits (type I syndrome). Zone 2 includes the deep branch of the ulnar nerve. Pathol-

ogy in zone 2 leads to motor deficits. Zone 3 includes the superficial branch of the ulnar nerve, which contains primarily sensory fibers. Therefore, patients (type III syndrome) present with sensory deficits.

Injury or compression to the ulnar nerve may be difficult to detect clinically.[4,5] Also, symptoms from ulnar nerve compression at the elbow (cubital tunnel syndrome) may be difficult to separate from nerve compression at the wrist.[41,48]

Ulnar nerve injury or compression may be related to blunt trauma (Fig. 9-16), fractures on the ulnar side of

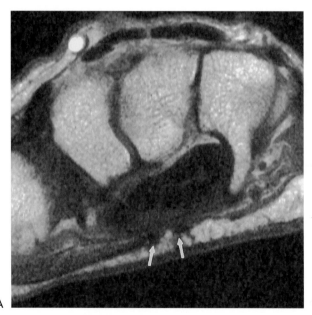

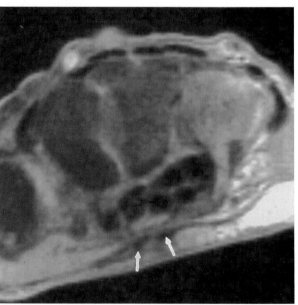

A   B

FIGURE 9-14. Axial T1- **(A)** and fast spin echo T2- **(B)** weighted images demonstrate an incomplete repair with scarring at the operative site *(arrow)* and no volar displacement of the retinacular fragments or palmar displacement of the carpal tunnel contents.

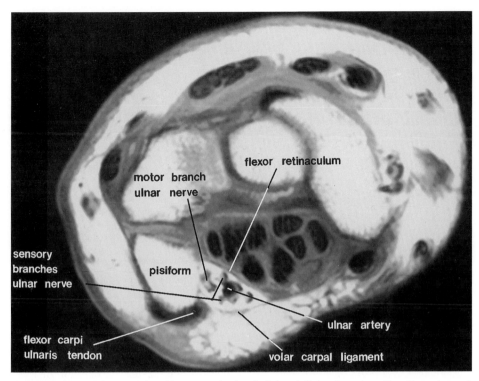

FIGURE 9-15. Axial T1-weighted image at the level of the pisiform demonstrating Guyon's canal.

the wrist, arthropathy with calcifications near the pisotriquetral joint, anomalous muscles, vascular anomalies, and soft-tissue masses.[2,4,48,58] Soft-tissue masses in Guyon's canal are uncommon.[5,6] Lesions reported include ganglion cysts (most common) (Fig. 9-17), lipomas, giant cell tumors, posttraumatic neuromas, neurofibromas, and intraneural cysts.[2,4,6,48,58]

Routine radiography may be adequate for detection of fractures or calcifications in the canal.[5,48] Ultrasonography and CT may also be useful.[2,48] However, we prefer MRI in most cases due to the superior soft-tissue contrast.

Axial MR images using the same approaches described for evaluating carpal tunnel syndrome can be employed.[5] Contrast enhancement may be useful, but motion studies are less commonly required.[5] MRI can clearly define the anatomy, pathology in the nerve or perineural tissues, and muscle involvement (Figs. 9-15 to 9-17).[4,5,33] If the results of MRI studies are normal, nerve conduction studies to exclude cubital tunnel syndrome or imaging of the elbow should be considered.[4,5]

Treatment varies depending on the etiologic factors. Patients with blunt trauma or overuse are treated conservatively

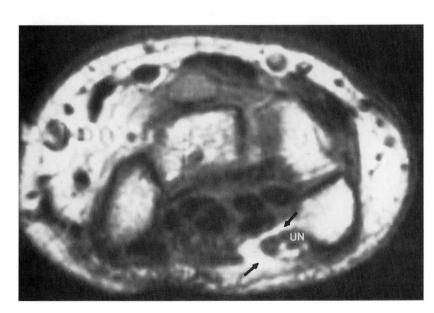

FIGURE 9-16. Axial T2-weighted image demonstrating increased signal intensity *(arrows)* surrounding Guyon's canal due to posttraumatic inflammation. UN, ulnar nerve.

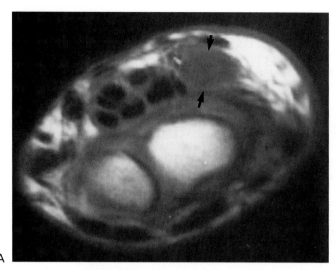
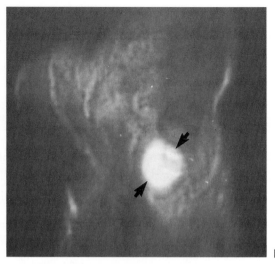

FIGURE 9-17. Axial T1- **(A)** and coronal T2- **(B)** weighted images demonstrating a ganglion cyst *(arrows)* compressing the ulnar nerve.

with rest and splinting. Surgical decompression is most effective when an intra- or extraneural etiology such as a soft-tissue mass, can be defined.[4,5,48]

Miscellaneous Syndromes

Other nerve syndromes may also affect the hand and wrist. These occur infrequently in comparison with median and ulnar nerve disorders. Anterior interosseous nerve syndrome is an example. The anterior interosseous nerve is a branch of the median nerve that comes off 2 to 8 cm below the medial epicondyle.[47] The anterior interosseous nerve passes distally in the anterior compartment. This motor nerve supplies the flexor pollicis longus, the flexor digitorum profundus of the index and middle fingers, and the pronator quadratus (Fig. 9-1).[17,47] The syndrome results in weakness of the muscles supplied by the nerve, but sensation is normal. Clinically, the condition may be difficult to differentiate from tendon ruptures in the hand. The flexor pollicis longus is often the weakest, suggesting rupture of its tendon.[17] Nerve conduction studies may be diagnostic. However, abnormal signal intensity in the muscles on MR images usually appear before electromyographic findings.[17,28,36]

The etiology may be related to self-limited neuritis, trauma (fracture, laceration), entrapment by soft-tissue masses, the tendinous origin of the pronator teres, enlargement of biceps bursae, or thrombosis of ulnar collateral vessels.[17,44]

Magnetic resonance imaging should include axial T1- and fat-suppressed T2-weighted or short T1 inversion recovery (STIR) images.[5,17] Muscles supplied by the anterior interosseous nerve demonstrate increased signal intensity on T2-weighted and STIR sequences (Fig. 9-18). In this setting, imaging should be extended to the level of the elbow to evaluate the cause more completely.

Treatment is conservative if no underlying etiologic factors can be defined. Surgical exploration is indicated when entrapment or a soft-tissue abnormality is identified.[17,44]

Petiot et al.[37] described a slowly progressive muscle atrophy involving both hands that resulted in muscle weakness and atrophy over a 20-year period. The extent of involvement and bilateral involvement excluded Hirayama's disease (unilateral atrophy that stabilizes after 2 years) and amyotrophic lateral sclerosis.[37] MR images of the cervical spine show increased signal intensity in the anterior cord and muscle atrophy with fatty replacement or increased signal intensity is evident in the hands.[37]

Radial nerve branch compression is rare but can occur with dorsal ganglion cysts. When evaluating nerve compression syndromes in the hand and wrist, one must consider

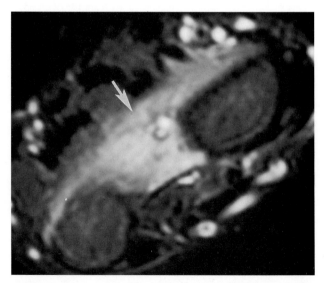

FIGURE 9-18. Anterior interosseous nerve syndrome. Axial, fat-suppressed, T2-weighted fast spin echo image demonstrates increased signal intensity in the pronator muscle *(arrow)*.

more proximal pathology in the cubital fossa or brachial plexus.[5,48]

REFERENCES

1. Albornoz MA, Mezgarzedeh M, Neumann CH, et al. Granulomatous tenosynovitis: a rare manifestation of tuberculosis. Clin Rheumatol 1998;17:166–169.
2. Anderson M, Kaplan PA, Dussault RG, et al. Magnetic resonance imaging of the wrist. Curr Probl Diagn Radiol 1998;Nov/Dec:187–229.
3. Bak L, Bak S, Gaster P, et al. MR imaging of the wrist in carpal tunnel syndrome. Acta Radiologica 1997;38:1050–1052.
4. Barberie JE, Connell DG, Munk PL, et al. Ulnar nerve injuries of the hand producing intrinsic muscle denervation on magnetic resonance imaging. Australasian Radiol 1999;43:355–357.
5. Berquist TH. MRI of the musculoskeletal system, 4th ed. Philadelphia: Lippincott Williams & Wilkins, 2001:773–841.
6. Binkovitz LA, Berquist TH, McLeod RA, et al. Masses of hand and wrist: detection and characterization using MR imaging. AJR 1989;154:223–236.
7. Binkovitz LA, Ehman RL, Cahill DR, et al. Magnetic resonance imaging of the wrist: normal cross-sectional imaging and selected abnormal cases. Radiographics 1988;8:1171–1202.
8. Brahme SK, Hodler J, Braun RM, et al. Dynamic MR imaging of carpal tunnel syndrome. Skel Radiol 1997;26:482–487.
9. Chen CKH, Chung CB, Yeh L-R, et al. Carpal tunnel syndrome caused by tophaceous gout. CT and MR imaging features in 20 patients. AJR 2000;175:655–659.
10. Cobb TK, Dalley BK, Posteraro RH, et al. Establishment of carpal contents/carpal canal ratio by means of magnetic resonance imaging. J Hand Surg 1992;17A:843–849.
11. Cobb TK, Dalley BK, Posteraro RH, et al. Anatomy of the flexor retinaculum. J Hand Surg 1993;18A:91–99.
12. Cobb TK, Carmichael SW, Cooney WP. Guyon's canal revisited: an anatomic study of the carpal ulnar neurovascular space. J Hand Surg 1996;21A:861–869.
13. Cobb TK, Bond JR, Cooney WP, et al. Assessment of the ratio of carpal contents to carpal volume in patients with carpal tunnel syndrome: a preliminary report. J Hand Surg 1997;22A:635–639.
14. Cooney WP. Vascular and neurological anatomy of the wrist. In: Cooney WP, Linscheid RL, Dobyns JH, eds. The wrist: diagnosis and operative treatment. St Louis: Mosby, 1998:106–123.
15. DiMarcangelo MJ, Smith PA. Use of magnetic resonance imaging to diagnose common wrist disorders. JAOA 2000;4:228–231.
16. Gelberman RH, Eaton R, Uibaniak JR. Peripheral nerve compression. J Bone Joint Surg 1993;75A:1854–1878.
17. Grainger AJ, Campbell RSD, Stothard J. Anterior interosseous nerve syndrome: appearance at MR imaging in 3 cases. Radiology 1998;208:381–384.
18. Greening J, Smart S, Leary R, et al. Reduced movement of median nerve in carpal tunnel during wrist flexion in patients with nonspecific arm pain. Lancet 1999;354:217–218.
19. Hayman LA, Duncan G, Chiou-tan FY, et al. Sectional neuroanatomy of the upper limb: III. Forearm and hand. J Comput Assist Tomogr 2001;25:322–325.
20. Healy C, Watson JD, Longstaff A, et al. Magnetic resonance imaging of the carpal tunnel. J Hand Surg 1990;15B:243–248.
21. Hoffman KL, Bergman AG, Hoffman DK, et al. Tuberculosis tenosynovitis of the flexor tendons of the wrist: MR imaging with pathologic correlation. Skel Radiol 1996;25:186–188.
22. Jarvik JG, Kliot M, Maravilla KR. MR nerve imaging of the hand and wrist. Hand Clin 2000;16:13–24.
23. Keir PJ, Wells R. Changes in geometry of finger flexor tendons in the carpal tunnel with wrist posture and tendon load: an MRI study on normal wrists. Clin Biomechan 1999;14:635–645.
24. Kleindienst A, Hanim B, Hildebrandt G, et al. Diagnosis and staging of carpal tunnel syndrome: comparison of magnetic resonance imaging and intra-operative findings. Acta Neurochir 1996;138:228–233.
25. Lanz U. Anatomic variations in the median nerve in the carpal tunnel. J Hand Surg 1977;2A:44–53.
26. Mäurer J, Bleschkowski A, Tempka A, et al. High resolution MR imaging of the carpal tunnel and wrist. Acta Radiol 2000;41:78–83.
27. Mesgarzedeh M, Schneck CE, Bonakdapour A, et al. Carpal tunnel: MR imaging: I. Normal anatomy. Radiology 1989;171:743–748.
28. Mesgarzedeh M, Schneck CE, Bonakdapour A, et al. Carpal tunnel: MR imaging: II. Carpal tunnel syndrome. Radiology 1989;171:749–754.
29. Mesgarzedeh M, Tiolo S, Schneck CD. Carpal tunnel syndrome: MR imaging diagnoses. Magn Reson Imaging Clin N Am 1995;3:249–264.
30. Meyer B-U, Röricht S, Schmitt R. Bilateral fibrolipomatous hamartoma of the median nerve with macrocheiria and late-onset nerve entrapment syndrome. Muscle and Nerve 1998;21:656–658.
31. Middleton WD, Kneeland JB, Kellman GM, et al. MR imaging of carpal tunnel: normal anatomy and preliminary findings in carpal tunnel syndrome. AJR 1987;148:307–316.
32. Nakamichi K, Tachkbana S. Unilateral carpal tunnel syndrome and space-occupying lesions. J Hand Surg 1993;18B:748–749.
33. Netcher D, Polsen C, Thornby J, et al. Anatomic delineation of the ulnar nerve and ulnar artery in relation to the carpal tunnel by axial magnetic resonance imaging scanning. J Hand Surg 1996;21A:273–276.
34. Netcher D, Mosharrofa A, Lee M, et al. Transverse carpal ligament: its effect on flexor tendon excursion, morphologic changes of the carpal canal and on pinch and grip strengths after open carpal tunnel release. Plastic Reconst Surg 1997;100:636–642.
35. Ogose A, Hotta J, Morita T, et al. Tumors of the peripheral nerves: correlation of symptoms, clinical signs imaging features and histologic diagnosis. Skel Radiol 1999;28:123–128.
36. Park TA, Welshofer JA, Dzwierzynski WW, et al. Median pseudoneuroapraxia at the wrist: reassessment of palmar stimulation of the recurrent median nerve. Arch Phys Med Rehab 2001;82:190–197.
37. Petiot P, Gonon V, Froment JC, et al. Slowly progressive spinal muscular atrophy of the hands (O'Sullivan-McLeod syndrome): clinical and magnetic resonance imaging presentation. J Neurol 2000;247:654–655.
38. Phalen GS. Carpal tunnel syndrome: clinical evaluation of 598 hands. Clin Orthop 1972;83:29–40.
39. Pierre-Jerome C, Bekklund SI, Husby G, et al. MRI anatomic variants of the wrist in women. Surg Radiol Anat 1996;18:37–41.
40. Pierre-Jerome C, Bekklund SI, Nordstrom R. Quantitative MRI analysis of anatomic dimension of the carpal tunnel in women. Surg Radiol Anat 1997;19:31–34.
41. Plancher KD, Peterson RK, Steichen JB. Compression neuropathies and tendinopathies in athletic elbow and wrist. Clin Sports Med 1996;15:331–371.
42. Propeck T, Quinn TJ, Jacobson JA, et al. Sonographic and MR imaging of bifid median nerve with anatomic and histologic correlation. AJR 2000;175:1721–1726.

43. Radack DM, Schweitzer ME, Taras J. Carpal tunnel syndrome: are the MR findings a result of population selection bias? AJR 1997;169:1649–1653.

44. Rask MR. Anterior interosseous nerve entrapment (Liloh-Nevin syndrome). Clin Orthop 1979;142:176–181.

45. Rempel D, Dahlin L, Lindborg G. Pathophysiology of nerve compression syndromes: response of peripheral nerves to loading. J Bone Joint Surg 1999;18A:1600–1610.

46. Richman JA, Gelberman RH, Rydevik BL, et al. Carpal tunnel volume determination by magnetic resonance imaging three-dimensional reconstruction. J Hand Surg 1987;12A:712–717.

47. Rosse C, Rosse PC. Hollinghead's textbook of anatomy. Philadelphia: Lippincott–Raven Publishers, 1997:239–306.

48. Sakai K, Tsutsui T, Aoi M, et al. Ulnar neuropathy caused by a lipoma in Guyon's canal. Neurol Med Chir 2000;40:335–338.

49. Schuerrman AH, van Gils APG. Reversed palmaris longus muscle on MRI: a report of four cases. Eur Radiol 2000;10:1242–1244.

50. Shum C, Parisien M, Strauch RJ, et al. The role of flexor tenosynovectomy in the operative treatment of carpal tunnel syndrome. J Bone Joint Surg 2002;84A:221–225.

51. Spinner RJ, Lins RE, Spinver M. Compression of the medial half of the deep branch of the ulnar nerve by an anomalous origin of the flexor digiti minimi. J Bone Joint Surg 1996;78A:427–430.

52. Sueyoski E, Uetani M, Hayaski K, et al. Tuberculous tenosynovitis of the wrist: MRI findings in three patients. Skel Radiol 1996;25:569–572.

53. Sugimoto H, Miyayi N, Ohsawa T. Carpal tunnel syndrome: evaluation of median nerve circulation with dynamic contrast enhanced MR imaging. Radiology 1994;190:459–466.

54. Szabo RM, Madison M. Carpal tunnel syndrome. Orthop Clin N Am 1992;23:103–109.

55. Timins ME. Muscular anatomic variants of the wrist and hand: findings on MR imaging. AJR 1999;172:1397–1401.

56. Zagnoli F, Andre V, LeDreff P, et al. Idiopathic carpal tunnel syndrome: clinical, electrodiagnostic, and magnetic resonance imaging correlations. Rev Rheum 1999;66:192–200.

57. Zeiss J, Guilliam-Haidet L. MR demonstration of anomalous muscle of the volar aspect of the wrist and forearm. Clin Imaging 1996;20:219–221.

58. Zeiss J, Jakab E, Khimji T, et al. The ulnar tunnel of the wrist (Guyon's canal): normal MR anatomy and variants. AJR 1992;158:1081–1085.

59. Zeiss J, Skie M, Ebraheim N, et al. Anatomic relations between the median nerve and flexor tendons in the carpal tunnel: MR evaluation on normal volunteers. AJR 1989;153:533–536.

MISCELLANEOUS CONDITIONS

THOMAS H. BERQUIST

There are numerous conditions that either affect the hand and wrist uncommonly or in which the role of magnetic resonance imaging (MRI) is not clearly defined.[2,13] Certain conditions are uncommon in the hand and wrist but MR features are defined. An example is pigmented villonodular synovitis. The MR features are well defined in the literature, but the condition is uncommon in the hand and wrist, especially in children.[4,12] Pigmented villonodular synovitis was discussed in Chapter 6 and will not be reviewed in this section.

REFLEX SYMPATHETIC DYSTROPHY

Reflex sympathetic dystrophy (RSD) is a distinct entity that most commonly involves the shoulder and hand. Though the condition is usually associated with trauma, the true etiology is unknown. Neurologic, vascular, and musculoskeletal disorders of any type may be related.[20,25] Shoulder-hand syndrome involves both structures with sparing of the elbow. This syndrome usually follows trauma, shoulder tendonitis, or myocardial infarction.[25]

Patients with RSD in the hand present with stiffness, swelling, pain, vasomotor changes, and hyperesthesia.[20] Onset of symptoms may occur weeks to months after the inciting event.[25] Clinical diagnosis may be difficult.[11,25] Symptoms may resolve gradually or remain for years.[20] Differential diagnosis include transient migratory osteoporosis, regional osteoporosis, rheumatoid arthritis, infection, and pigmented villonodular synovitis.[20,25]

Radiographs may demonstrate soft-tissue swelling and osteopenia. The latter is most obvious in juxta-articular regions. Cortical resorption may result in longitudinal lucent tunnels.[20,25] Technetium-99m methylene diphosphonate (MDP) scans, obtained using three-phase technique, demonstrate increased flow and increased tracer in juxta-articular regions on delayed images.[2,25]

Magnetic resonance features of RSD have not been clearly defined resulting in decreased specificity.[14,20] Features described include skin thickening that enhances after intravenous gadolinium on fat-suppressed T1-weighted images,

juxta-articular enhancement or increased signal intensity on T2-weighted images, and joint effusions.[2,11] The presence of joint effusion increases the sensitivity for diagnosis of RSD from 60% to 91%.[20]

SYNOVIAL CHONDROMATOSIS/ OSTEOCHONDROMATOSIS

This condition is the result of cartilaginous, osteoid, or osteocartilaginous metaplasia of the synovium. The etiology is unknown.[20-23] The knee, hip, and elbow are most commonly involved. Males outnumber females 2:1. The majority of patients are in the 30- to 50-year age range. The disorder has been reported from infancy to 70+ years of age. Chondromatosis or osteochondromatosis is rare in the hand and wrist. Patients tend to be older (mean age 50 years).[23] The condition is typically monoarticular. The distal radioulnar joint is commonly involved.[21] The tendon sheaths of the hand and wrist account for nearly half of the cases reported.[23]

Milgram[17] described three phases of this progressive ongoing process. The first phase is intrasynovial proliferation. Phase 2 is active synovial disease with loose bodies, and phase 3 is inactive synovial disease with loose bodies.[17,21,23]

Patients present with progressive swelling, pain, and decreased range of motion of the involved joint.[20,21] Differential diagnosis varies with location. However, degenerative joint disease with fragments in the joint space, osteochondritis dissecans, osteochondral fractures, and joint neuropathy may mimic osteochondromatosis.[23]

Routine radiographs demonstrate soft-tissue swelling, multiple dense shadows (millimeters to centimeters in size), bone erosion, and varying degrees of calcification or ossification in or about the joints or along the tendon sheaths of the hand and wrist.[2,20]

Early synovial changes due to synovial proliferation may be evident on arthrograms or MR images.[2,8,26] Arthrograms demonstrate synovial irregularity and loose bodies. Similar features can be seen with other causes of chronic synovitis with synovial frond formation or with rice bodies in patients with tuberculosis.[2]

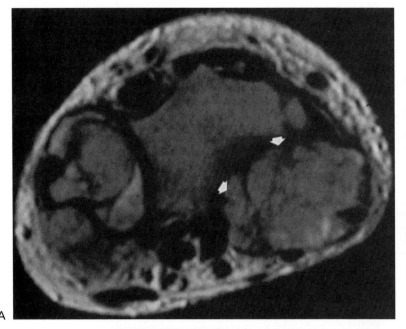

A

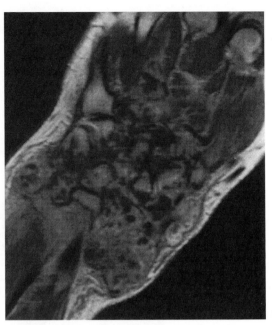

B

FIGURE 10-1. Axial **(A)** and coronal **(B)** T1-weighted images demonstrate synovial proliferation with multiple low-intensity loose bodies and radial erosion *(arrows)* due to synovial chondromatosis. (From Rompen JC, Ham SJ, Molenaar WM, et al. Synovial chondromatosis of the wrist and hand: a case report. Acta Orthop Scand 1999;70:627–629.)

Magnetic resonance imaging can be performed using conventional pulse sequences or with intravenous or intra-articular gadolinium.[2,8,21] T2-weighted spin echo or fast spin echo sequences may demonstrate significant joint effusions in early or phase 1 disease.[21] Active synovial disease enhances and foci of intermediate or low-density metaplasia may be evident depending on the cartilaginous, osseous, or calcified nature of the synovium. The appearance of loose bodies also varies with their histology. Loose bodies may have a high intensity outer cartilage layer with intermediate to high signal intensity centrally.[8] Some loose bodies are low signal intensity on T1- and T2-weighted sequences (Fig. 10-1).[2,8]

Management of synovial chondromatosis or osteochondromatosis varies with the phase. Phase 1 disease is managed with synovectomy, and phase 2 disease with synovectomy and loose body removal. Phase 3 disease (no active synovial disease) is managed with loose-body removal.[22] Baseline postoperative MR studies with intravenous gadolinium

are useful as reoccurrence takes place in 18% to 24% of cases.[23]

MARROW EDEMA

Bone marrow edema results from increased water content from a number of etiologies. A single structure or multiple osseous structures may be involved (Table 10-1).[1]

TABLE 10-1. BONE MARROW EDEMA ETIOLOGIC FACTORS[1,2,8,26]

Avascular necrosis
Fracture
Infection
Neoplasms
Reflex sympathetic dystrophy
Regional osteoporosis
Transient migratory osteoporosis

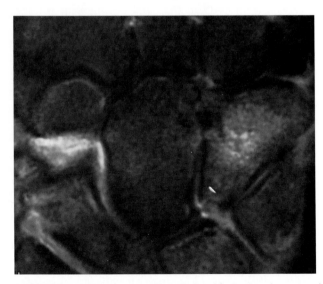

FIGURE 10-2. Fat-suppressed T2-weighted fast spin echo coronal image demonstrates increased signal intensity due to edema in the proximal carpal row and hamate.

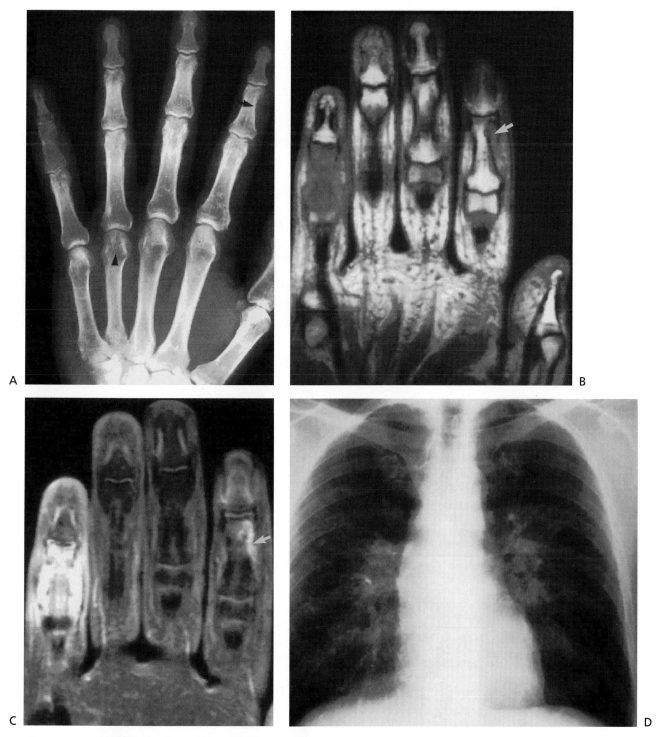

FIGURE 10-3. Sarcoidosis. **(A)** Posteroanterior radiograph of the left hand demonstrates trabecular and cortical destruction of the fifth middle phalanx and a small defect in the index finger *(arrow)* and fourth metacarpal *(arrowhead)*. Coronal T1- **(B)** and T2-weighted **(C)** images demonstrate low signal intensity **(B)** and high signal intensity **(C)** changes in the involved phalanx and index finger *(arrow)*. Chest radiograph **(D)** demonstrates hilar adenopathy and pulmonary infiltrates. (From Bigattni D, Daenen B, Dondelinger RF. Osseous sarcoidosis. JBR-BTR 1999;82:108.)

When radiographs are normal or equivocal, MR images may demonstrate not only the edema but also the underlying etiologic factors.[2,8]

Alam et al.[1] reviewed 519 patients and found marrow edema in 187 (36%). The majority of the cases were related to arthropathies (50.5%), fracture (36%), or avascular necrosis (13.5%).[1]

Marrow edema is low signal intensity on T1- and high signal intensity on T2-weighted sequences (Fig. 10-2). Enhancement occurs after intravenous gadolinium if flow is intact.[2] Bone marrow edema in the lunate, scaphoid, and capitate may represent a stress fracture or a bone bruise. Follow-up evaluation is warranted as the edema may also represent the earliest phase of avascular necrosis.

SARCOIDOSIS

Sarcoidosis is a granulomatous disease of unknown etiology. Multiple organ systems, including the musculoskeletal system, are involved with noncaseating granulomas.[20] Pulmonary involvement with hilar and paratracheal adenopathy and/or lung involvement occurs in 90% of patients. Ocular involvement occurs in 25%, skin disease (erythema nodosum) in 10% to 60%, and osseous involvement in about 5% of patients.[3,20] Osseous lesions are asymmetric, with involvement of the distal and middle phalanges and metacarpals occurring most frequently.[3,19]

Patients present with malaise, weight loss, and hepatosplenomegaly. Osseous lesions may be asymptomatic.[20] Routine radiographs demonstrate permeative changes in the marrow and cortex to create a lace-like appearance. Focal lytic lesions are also common. Soft-tissue swelling occurs in some cases. However, joint involvement and periosteal reaction are unusual.[3,19]

Magnetic resonance images show areas of increased signal intensity on T2-weighted and low intensity on T1-weighted images (Fig. 10-3). These changes may be diffuse with similar changes in the soft tissues when a permeative pattern is present or focal with smaller lytic areas.[3] Tuberculosis, fungal infections, and multiple enchondromas may have a similar appearance.[20]

MADELUNG'S DEFORMITY

Madelung's deformity occurs with bowing and shortening of the distal radius, with the ulna remaining straight and, therefore, longer.[5,20] Isolated Madelung's is frequently bilateral and three to five times more common in females.[20] The deformity may result from multiple factors. Madelung's may be seen with dyschondrosteosis, hereditary multiple exostoses, Turner's syndrome, or following infection, trauma, or tumor development.[18]

Most patients present as adolescents or in childhood.[5,18] Pain, deformity, and decreased range of motion are common.[5,20]

Radiographs (Fig. 10-4) demonstrate bowing and shortening of the radius with a straight longer ulna and prominent ulnar head.[5,20] The radial bowing is typically 8 to 10°.[5] In patients with dyschondrosteosis, the radius and ulna may be thicker and the bowing more severe (15 to 17°).[5] The carpal angle (normal 130 to 137°) is reduced, resulting in a wedge appearance of the carpus.[20]

Magnetic resonance images demonstrate similar features. Coronal, sagittal, and axial image planes should be obtained (Fig. 10-5). T2-weighted or T2* gradient echo sequences are

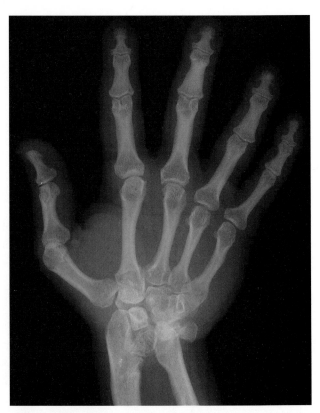

FIGURE 10-4. Posteroanterior radiograph in a patient with Madelung's deformity.

best for evaluating the growth plates. T1-weighted sequences are adequate for osseous anatomy. Cook et al.[5] noted loss of the lunate facet on the radial articular surface or axial images. Physeal bars were noted in the distal volar radius. These bars measured up to 17 mm on sagittal and 16 to 20 mm on coronal images. The carpal angle averaged 93° on coronal images (normal 130 to 137°) (Fig. 10-5).[5,17]

MYOSITIS OSSIFICANS

Myositis ossificans is heterotopic ossification in the muscles, fascia, or tendons.[20] The condition is almost always related to trauma (75%).[15,16,20] Lesions are most common in the large muscles of the lower extremities (80%) but may also occur in other locations.[15,16] Myositis ossificans is rare in the hand and wrist.[9,10,16]

Patients present with a soft-tissue mass, pain, and tenderness over the involved region.[16] Radiographs demonstrate faint peripheral calcification by 2 to 6 weeks. This gradually matures and becomes more dense over 5 to 6 months.[15,27]

Magnetic resonance features vary with the maturity of the lesion. Early lesions are high signal intensity on T2-weighted sequences and isointense compared with muscle on T1-weighted sequences.[16] There is usually a thin, low-intensity rim. Fluid-fluid levels may be seen from previous hemorrhage.[27]

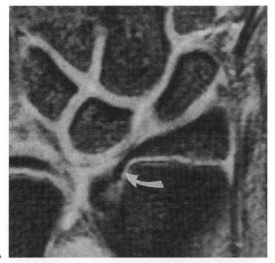

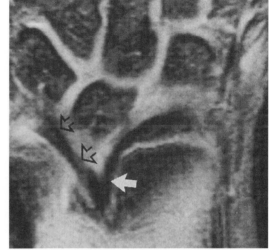

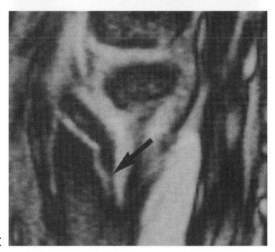

FIGURE 10-5. Madelung's deformity. **A:** Coronal GRE image demonstrates wrapping of the radial physis over the metaphysis *(arrow)*. **B:** A more anterior coronal image demonstrates more severe wrapping of the physeal plate. A portion of the fibrous bar is evident *(white arrow)* as well as a hypertropic anomalous volar radiotriquetral ligament *(double open arrows)*. **C:** Sagittal gradient recalled echo image demonstrates the junction of the epiphysis and physeal bar *(arrow)*. (From Cook PA, Yu JS, Wiand W, et al. Madelung deformity in skeletally immature patients: morphologic assessment using radiography, CT and MRI. J Comput Assist Tomogr 1996;20:505–511.)

Mature lesions have an inhomogeneous well-defined rim on all pulse sequences. There are typically areas of mature fat, marrow, and hemosiderin. Active lesions enhance with intravenous gadolinium.[15] Treatment is local excision.[15,16]

MICROGEODE SYNDROME

The etiology of microgeode syndrome of the phalanges is unknown. However, it is related to cold exposure and frostbite. Patients present with pain and swelling in the fingers. The middle phalanges of the index and middle fingers are most commonly involved. Multiple lesions occur in 50% of cases, and the condition is bilateral in about 33% of patients.[7]

Histologically there is mixed bone necrosis and repair. The condition is typically self-limited with resolution in 2 to 3 months.[24]

Clinical examination and radiographs may be diagnostic. Radiographs demonstrate small lucanae in the phalanges.[7] Focal or defuse areas of low intensity on T1- and high intensity on T2-weighted sequences is apparent in the involved phalanges and adjacent soft tissues (Fig. 10-6). As expected, the involved tissues enhance following intravenous gadolin-ium. Multiple lesions and bilateral involvement assist in excluding infection or neoplasm, which could be considered in the differential diagnosis.[7,24]

TISSUE OVERGROWTH SYNDROMES

There are a number of tissue overgrowth syndromes that may involve the hand and wrist. These include macrodactyly, angiolipomatosis, Klippel-Trenaunay-Weber syndrome, and macrodystrophia lipomatosis (Fig. 10-7).[6] Congenital disorders produce asymmetry and bone and soft-tissue hypertrophy due to disordered embryogenesis.

T1- and T2-weighted MR images may define the abnormality when clinical or radiographic findings are equivocal.[6] Vascular lesions can be more easily defined using contrast-enhanced MR angiography.[2]

FOREIGN BODIES

The presence of soft-tissue foreign bodies in the hand is common. Opaque foreign bodies can be localized with

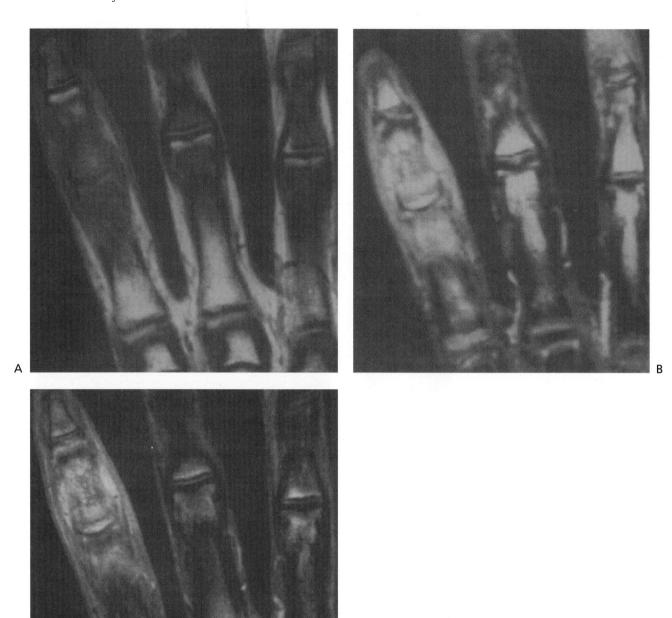

FIGURE 10-6. Microgeode syndrome. **A:** Coronal T1-weighted image demonstrates low signal intensity in the second through fourth phalanges. **B:** Short TI inversion recovery (STIR) image shows increased signal intensity in the same locations. **C:** Contrast-enhanced T1-weighted image shows marked enhancement of the middle phalanx of the index finger. (From Fugita A, Sugimoto H, Kikkawa I, et al. Phalangeal microgeode syndrome: findings on MR imaging. AJR 1999;173:711–712.)

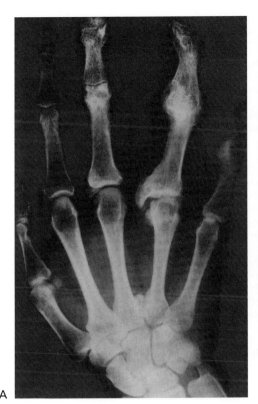
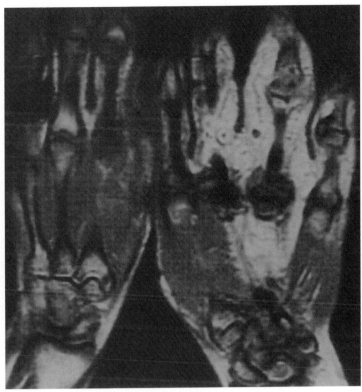

A   B

FIGURE 10-7. Macrodystrophia lipomatosa. **A:** Radiograph demonstrates overgrowth of the third through fifth fingers. **B:** Coronal T1-weighted MR image demonstrates fatty proliferation. (From D'Costa H, Hunter JD, O'Sullivan G, et al. Magnetic resonance imaging of macromelia and macrodactyly. Br J Radiol 1996;69:502–507.)

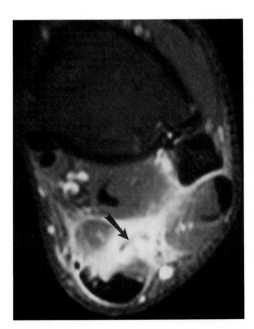

FIGURE 10-8. Contrast-enhanced image demonstrates soft-tissue inflammation with a rose thorn *(arrow).*

routine radiography. Nonopaque foreign bodies can present a challenge. Ultrasound and MRI have been selected to localize foreign bodies and define areas of associated infection more frequently in recent years.[2,26] Foreign bodies appear as low-intensity nonanatomic structures on MR images.[26] Three-dimensional gradient echo images are most useful for detection and anatomic localization. Gadolinium is also useful to enhance inflamed tissues and increase the conspicuity of the foreign body (Fig. 10-8).[26]

REFERENCES

1. Alam F, Schweitzer ME, Li X-X, et al. Frequency and spectrum of abnormalities in the bone marrow of the wrist: MR imaging findings. Skel Radiol 1999;28:312–317.
2. Berquist TH. MRI of the musculoskeletal system, 4th ed. Philadelphia: Lippincott Williams & Wilkins, 2001:1029–1068.
3. Bigattini D, Daenen B, Dondelinger RF. Osseous sarcoidosis. J. Belge de Radiologie–Belgisch Tijdschrift/voor Radiologie 1999; 82:108.
4. Carpintero P, Serrano J, Garcia-Frasquet A. Pigmented villonodular synovitis of the wrist invading bone: a report of 2 cases. Acta Orthop Scand 2000;71:424–426.
5. Cook PA, Yu JS, Wiand W, et al. Madelung deformity in skeletally immature patients: morphologic assessment using radiography, CT and MRI. J Comput Assist Tomogr 1996;20:505–511.
6. D'Costa H, Hunter JD, O'Sullivan G, et al. Magnetic resonance imaging of macromelia and macrodactyly. Br J Radiol 1996;69:502–507.

7. Fujita A, Sugimoto H, Kikikawa I, et al. Phalangeal microgeode syndrome: findings on MR imaging. AJR 1999;173:711–712.
8. Gilula LA, Yin Y. Imaging of the wrist and hand. Philadelphia: WB Saunders, 1996.
9. Goldman AB. Myositis ossificans circumscripta: a benign lesion with a malignant differential diagnosis. AJR 1976;126:32–40.
10. Goto H, Hatori M, Kokubun S, et al. Myositis ossificans in the tip of the thumb. A case report. Tohoku J Exp Med 1998;184:67–72.
11. Graif M, Schweitzer ME, Marks B, et al. Synovial effusion in reflex sympathetic dystrophy: an additional sign for diagnosis and staging. Skel Radiol 1998;27:262–265.
12. Hoeffel JC, Mainard L, Champignuelle J, et al. Pigmented villonodular synovitis of the wrist in childhood. Clin Pediatr 1997;36:423–426.
13. Kontoyianni A, Maragou M, Alvonou E, et al. Unilateral distal extremity swelling with pitting edema in giant cell arteritis. Clin Rheumatol 1999;18:82–84.
14. Koch E, Hofer HO, Sialer G, et al. Failure of MR imaging to detect reflex sympathetic dystrophy of the extremities. AJR 1991;156:113–115.
15. Kransdorf MJ, Meis JM, Jelinek JS. Myositis ossificans: MR appearance with radiologic–pathologic correlation. AJR 1991;157:1243–1248.
16. Kransdorf MJ, Berquist TH. Musculoskeletal neoplasms. In: Berquist TH, ed. MRI of the musculoskeletal system, 4th ed. Philadelphia: Lippincott Williams & Wilkins, 2001:842–955.
17. Milgram JW. Synovial osteochondromatosis: a histopathologic study of thirty cases. J Bone Joint Surg 1977;59A:792–801.
18. Neilsen JB. Madelung's deformity: a follow-up of 26 cases and a review of the literature. Acta Orthop Scand 1997;48:379–384.
19. Posner MA, Melendez E, Steiner G. Solitary osseous sarcoidosis in a finger. J Hand Surg 1991;16A:827–831.
20. Resnick D. Bone and joint imaging, 2nd ed. Philadelphia: WB Saunders, 1996.
21. Rogachefsky RA, Zlatkin MB, Greene TL. Synovial chondromatosis of the distal radioulnar joint: A case report. J Hand Surg 1997;22A:1093–1097.
22. Rompen JC, Ham SJ, Molenaar WM, et al. Synovial chondromatosis of the hand and wrist: a case report. Acta Orthop Scand 1999;70:627–629.
23. Roulot E, LeViet D. Primary osteochondromatosis of the hand and wrist. A report of a series of 21 cases and literature review. Rev Rheum 1999;66:256–266.
24. Sato K, Sugiura H, Aoki M. Transient phalangeal osteolysis (microgeode disease): report of a case involving the foot. J Bone Joint Surg 1995;77A:1888–1890.
25. Sintzoff S, Sintzoff S Jr, Stallenberg B, et al. Imaging of reflex sympathetic dystrophy. Hand Clin 1997;13:431–442.
26. Totterman SMS, Miller RJ. MRI of the wrist and hand. In: Gilula L, Yin Y, eds. Imaging of the wrist and hand. Philadelphia: WB Saunders, 1996:441–479.
27. Tsai JC, Dalinka MK, Fallon MD, et al. Fluid-fluid level: a nonspecific finding in tumors of bone and soft tissues. Radiology 1990;175:779–782.

SUBJECT INDEX

Note: Page numbers followed by f indicate figures; those followed by t indicate tables.